Abbreviations

D&C	dilatation and (sharp) curettage
D&E	dilatation and evacuation
EVA	electric vacuum aspiration
GMP	good manufacturing practice
GRADE	Grading of Recommendations Assessment, Development and Evaluation
hCG	human chorionic gonadotrophin
HIV	human immunodeficiency virus
HLD	high-level disinfection
ICPD	International Conference on Population and Development
IUD	intrauterine device
IV	intravenous
KCl	potassium chloride
LMP	last menstrual period
MVA	manual vacuum aspiration
NGO	nongovernmental organization
PG	prostaglandin
Rh	Rhesus (blood group)
RTI	reproductive tract infection
STI	sexually transmitted infection
UN	United Nations
UNFPA	United Nations Population Fund
UNPD	United Nations Population Division
USA	United States of America
WHO	World Health Organization

Definitions used in this document

- *Duration or gestational age of pregnancy (gestation)*: the number of days or weeks since the first day of the woman's last normal menstrual period (LMP) in women with regular cycles (for women with irregular cycles, the gestational age may need to be determined by physical or ultrasound examination). The first trimester is generally considered to consist of the first 12 or the first 14 weeks of pregnancy (see Table 1).

Table 1. Equivalent gestational ages in weeks and days during the first trimester

Weeks of gestation	Days of gestation
<1	0–6
1	7–13
2	14–20
3	21–27
4	28–34
5	35–41
6	42–48
7	49–55
8	56–62
9	63–69
10	70–76
11	77–83
12	84–90
13	91–97
14	98–104

Adapted from: *International statistical classification of diseases and health related problems, 10th revision – ICD-10*, Vol. 2, 2008 Edition. Geneva, World Health Organization, 2009.

- *Medical methods of abortion (medical abortion)*: use of pharmacological drugs to terminate pregnancy. Sometimes the terms "non-surgical abortion" or "medication abortion" are also used.

- *Menstrual regulation*: uterine evacuation without laboratory or ultrasound confirmation of pregnancy for women who report recent delayed menses.

- *Osmotic dilators:* short, thin rods made of seaweed (laminaria) or synthetic material. After placement in the cervical os, the dilators absorb moisture and expand, gradually dilating the cervix.

- *Routes of misoprostol administration:*

  - oral – pills are swallowed immediately;

  - buccal – pills are placed between the cheek and gums and swallowed after 30 minutes;

  - sublingual – pills are placed under the tongue and swallowed after 30 minutes;

  - vaginal – pills are placed in the vaginal fornices (deepest portions of the vagina) and the woman is instructed to lie down for 30 minutes.

- *Surgical methods of abortion (surgical abortion)*: use of transcervical procedures for terminating pregnancy, including vacuum aspiration and dilatation and evacuation (D&E). (See Chapter 2, Section 2.2.4 for a more detailed description of methods of surgical abortion.)

Human Rights terminology

- *International human rights treaty:* also sometimes called a Covenant or a Convention, is adopted by the international community of States, normally at the United Nations General Assembly. Each treaty sets out a range of human rights, and corresponding obligations which are legally binding on States that have ratified the treaty. Annex 7 includes a list of these treaties.

Safe abortion:
technical and policy guidance
for health systems

Second edition

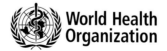

World Health Organization

Acknowledgements

WHO is grateful for the technical contributions of the external experts who participated in the initial online consultation, the technical consultation and the review of this guideline.
(Details of participants and additional external reviewers are provided in Annex 4.)

Funding source

The development of these guidelines was supported by the UNDP/UNFPA/WHO/World Bank Special Programme of Research, Development and Research Training in Human Reproduction (HRP).

WHO Library Cataloguing-in-Publication Data

Safe abortion: technical and policy guidance for health systems – 2nd ed.

    1.Abortion, Induced - methods 2.Abortion, Induced - standards. 3.Prenatal
    care - organization and administration 4.Prenatal care - standards
    5.Maternal welfare 6.Health policy 7.Guidelines. I.World Health Organization.

    ISBN 978 92 4 154843 4   (NLM classification: WQ 440)

- *Treaty monitoring body:* each of the international human rights treaties is monitored by a designated treaty monitoring body (see Annex 7). The treaty monitoring bodies are committees composed of independent experts. Their main function is to monitor the States' compliance with the treaty in question, including through the examination of State reports.

- *General comments/recommendations:* a treaty monitoring body's interpretation of the content of human rights provisions on thematic issues or its methods of work. General comments seek to clarify the reporting duties of State parties with respect to certain provisions and suggest approaches to implementing treaty provisions.

- *Concluding observations:* following submission of a State report and a constructive dialogue with the State party to the particular convention, treaty monitoring bodies issue concluding observations to the reporting State, which are compiled in an annual report and sent to the United Nations General Assembly.

- *Regional human rights treaties:* States adopted human rights treaties in Africa, the Americas, Europe and the Middle East. Regional human rights bodies, such as the African Union, the Organization of American States, the Council of Europe, the European Union, and the League of Arab States monitor States' compliance with the treaties. To date, there are no regional human rights treaties in South-East Asia or the Western Pacific. Annex 7 includes a list of regional human rights treaties.

- *Human rights standards:* the meaning and scope of human rights as interpreted and applied by the human rights bodies tasked with this work, e.g. international, regional and national courts, and human rights committees.

CONTENTS

EXECUTIVE SUMMARY

Over the past two decades, the health evidence, technologies and human rights rationale for providing safe, comprehensive abortion care have evolved greatly. Despite these advances, an estimated 22 million abortions continue to be performed unsafely each year, resulting in the death of an estimated 47 000 women and disabilities for an additional 5 million women (1). Almost every one of these deaths and disabilities could have been prevented through sexuality education, family planning, and the provision of safe, legal induced abortion and care for complications of abortion. In nearly all developed countries, safe abortions are legally available upon request or under broad social and economic grounds, and services are generally easily accessible and available. In countries where induced abortion is legally highly restricted and/or unavailable, safe abortion has frequently become the privilege of the rich, while poor women have little choice but to resort to unsafe providers, causing deaths and morbidities that become the social and financial responsibility of the public health system.

In view of the need for evidence-based best practices for providing safe abortion care in order to protect the health of women, the World Health Organization (WHO) has updated its 2003 publication *Safe abortion: technical and policy guidance for health systems* (2). In this process, the WHO standards for guideline development have been followed, including: identification of priority questions and outcomes; retrieval, assessment and synthesis of evidence; formulation of recommendations; and planning for dissemination, implementation, impact evaluation and updating. For the clinical recommendations presented in Chapter 2, evidence profiles related to the prioritized questions were prepared, based upon recent systematic reviews, most of which are included in the *Cochrane Database of Systematic Reviews*. In addition, Chapters 1, 3 and 4 of the original 2003 publication were reviewed and updated to reflect the latest estimates on unsafe abortion worldwide, new literature on the topic of service delivery, and new developments in international, regional and national human rights law. A guideline development group, comprising members of an international panel of experts, reviewed and revised the draft recommendations based on the evidence profiles, through a participatory, consensus-driven process.

The target audience for this guidance is policy-makers, programme managers and providers of abortion care. The use of the clinical recommendations should be individualized to each woman, with emphasis on her clinical status and the specific method of abortion to be used, while considering each woman's preferences for care.

While legal, regulatory, policy and service-delivery contexts may vary from country to country, the recommendations and best practices described in this document aim to enable evidence-based decision-making with respect to safe abortion care. Details of their development and application of the quality of evidence grading are found under the Methods section, page 10. Box 1 presents the recommendations related to specific methods of surgical abortion, while Box 2 summarizes the recommendations for medical abortion. Box 3 addresses recommendations for the surgical or medical methods preferred beyond 12 weeks of gestation. Box 4 summarizes the recommendations related to clinical care prior to induced abortion, including consideration of cervical preparation, use of diagnostic ultrasonography, use of antibiotics and pain-management options. Box 5 summarizes the recommendations

related to post-abortion care, including initiation of contraception, treatment of incomplete abortion and whether there is a medical need for routine follow-up visits after induced abortion. Box 6 summarizes the main recommendations from Chapter 3 related to application of the clinical guidance in establishing and strengthening abortion services, including development of national standards and guidelines; training and equipping of service providers; assessing, prioritizing and financing of health-system needs; introducing and scaling-up of interventions; and monitoring and evaluation. Finally, Box 7 summarizes the main recommendations from Chapter 4 concerning legal, policy and human rights dimensions.

Members of the guideline development group noted important knowledge gaps that need to be addressed through primary research. Overall, the group placed a high value on research to demedicalize abortion care. Observations regarding the need for future research are presented in Annex 1.

BOX 1

Recommended methods for surgical abortion

Vacuum aspiration is the recommended technique of surgical abortion for pregnancies of up to 12 to 14 weeks of gestation. The procedure should not be routinely completed by sharp curettage. Dilatation and sharp curettage (D&C), if still practised, should be replaced by vacuum aspiration.

(Strength of recommendation: strong.
Quality of evidence based on randomized controlled trials: low to moderate.)

See also: Annex 5, Recommendation 1, page 113.

BOX 2

Recommended methods for medical abortion

The recommended method for medical abortion is mifepristone followed by misoprostol.

For pregnancies of gestational age up to 9 weeks (63 days)

The recommended method for medical abortion is mifepristone followed 1 to 2 days later by misoprostol.
[See notes below for dosages, and routes of administration.]

(Strength of recommendation: strong.
Quality of evidence based on randomized controlled trials: moderate.)

Dosages and routes of administration for mifepristone followed by misoprostol

Mifepristone should always be administered orally. The recommended dose is 200 mg.

Administration of **misoprostol** is recommended 1 to 2 days (24 to 48 hours) following ingestion of mifepristone.

- For vaginal, buccal or sublingual routes, the recommended dose of misoprostol is 800 µg.
- For oral administration, the recommended dose of misoprostol is 400 µg.
- With gestations up to **7 weeks** (49 days) misoprostol may be administered by vaginal, buccal, sublingual or oral routes. After 7 weeks of gestation, oral administration of misoprostol should *not* be used.
- With gestations up to **9 weeks** (63 days) misoprostol can be administered by vaginal, buccal or sublingual routes.

See also: Annex 5, Recommendation 2, page 113.

For pregnancies of gestational age between 9 and 12 weeks (63–84 days)

The recommended method for medical abortion is 200 mg mifepristone administered orally followed 36 to 48 hours later by 800 µg misoprostol administered vaginally. Subsequent misoprostol doses should be 400 µg, administered either vaginally or sublingually, every 3 hours up to four further doses, until expulsion of the products of conception.

(Strength of recommendation: weak.
Quality of evidence based on one randomized controlled trial and one observational study: low.)

See also: Annex 5, Recommendation 3, page 114.

For pregnancies of gestational age over 12 weeks (84 days)

The recommended method for medical abortion is 200 mg mifepristone administered orally followed 36 to 48 hours later by repeated doses of misoprostol.
[See notes below for dosages, and routes of administration of misoprostol.]

(Strength of recommendation: strong.
Quality of evidence based on randomized controlled trials: low to moderate.)

- With gestations between 12 and 24 weeks, the initial misoprostol dose following oral mifepristone administration may be either 800 µg administered vaginally or 400 µg administered orally. Subsequent misoprostol doses should be 400 µg, administered either vaginally or sublingually, every 3 hours up to four further doses.
- For pregnancies beyond 24 weeks, the dose of misoprostol should be reduced, due to the greater sensitivity of the uterus to prostaglandins, but the lack of clinical studies precludes specific dosing recommendations.

See also: Annex 5, Recommendation 6, page 115.

box 2 continued

Recommended methods for medical abortion

Where mifepristone is not available

For pregnancies of gestational age up to 12 weeks (84 days)

The recommended method of medical abortion is 800 μg of misoprostol administered by vaginal or sub-lingual routes. Up to three repeat doses of 800 μg can be administered at intervals of at least 3 hours, but for no longer than 12 hours.

(Strength of recommendation: strong.
Quality of evidence based on one randomized controlled trial: high.)

See also: Annex 5, Recommendation 4, page 115.

For pregnancies of gestational age over 12 weeks (84 days)

The recommended method of medical abortion is 400 μg of misoprostol administered vaginally or sub-lingually, repeated every 3 hours for up to five doses.

(Strength of recommendation: strong.
Quality of evidence based on one randomized controlled trial: low to moderate.)

- For pregnancies beyond 24 weeks, the dose of misoprostol should be reduced, due to the greater sensitivity of the uterus to prostaglandins, but the lack of clinical studies precludes specific dosing recommendations.

See also: Annex 5, Recommendation 6, pages 115 and 116.

BOX 3

Recommended methods of abortion for pregnancies of gestational age over 12 to 14 weeks

Dilatation and evacuation (D&E) and medical methods (mifepristone and misoprostol; misoprostol alone) are both recommended methods for abortion for gestation over 12 to 14 weeks. Facilities should offer at least one, and preferably both methods, if possible, depending on provider experience and the availability of training.

(Strength of recommendation: strong.
Quality of evidence based on randomized controlled trials: low.)

See also: Annex 5, Recommendation 5 page 115.

BOX 4

Recommendations for care preceding induced abortion

Cervical preparation

Prior to surgical abortion, cervical preparation is recommended for all women with a pregnancy over 12 to 14 weeks of gestation. Its use may be considered for women with a pregnancy of any gestational age.

(Strength of recommendation: strong.
Quality of evidence based on randomized controlled trials: low.)

- Any one of these methods of cervical preparation before surgical abortion in the first trimester is recommended:
  - oral mifepristone 200 mg (24 to 48 hours in advance); or
  - misoprostol 400 μg administered sublingually, 2 to 3 hours prior to the procedure; or
  - misoprostol 400 μg administered vaginally 3 hours prior to the procedure; or
  - laminaria placed intracervically 6 to 24 hours prior to the procedure.

(Strength of recommendation: strong.
Quality of evidence based on randomized controlled trials: low to moderate.)

See also: Annex 5, Recommendation 7, page 116.

All women undergoing dilatation and evacuation (D&E) with a pregnancy over 14 weeks of gestation should receive cervical preparation prior to the procedure.

(Strength of recommendation: strong.
Quality of the evidence based on randomized controlled trials: low to moderate.)

- The recommended methods of cervical preparation prior to dilatation and evacuation (D&E) after 14 weeks of gestation are osmotic dilators or misoprostol.

(Strength of recommendation: strong.
Quality of evidence based on randomized controlled trials: moderate.)

See also: Annex 5, Recommendation 8, page 117.

box 4 continued

Recommendations for care preceding induced abortion

Ultrasound scanning

Use of routine pre-abortion ultrasound scanning is not necessary.

(Strength of recommendation: strong.
Quality of evidence based on a randomized controlled trial and observational studies: very low.)

See also: Annex 5, Recommendation 12, page 118.

Prophylactic antibiotics

All women having surgical abortion, regardless of their risk of pelvic inflammatory infection, should receive appropriate prophylactic antibiotics pre- or peri-operatively.

(Strength of recommendation: strong.
Quality of evidence based on randomized controlled trials: moderate.)

See also: Annex 5, Recommendation 11, page 118.

For women having medical abortion, routine use of prophylactic antibiotics is not recommended.

(Strength of recommendation: strong.
Quality of evidence based on one observational trial: very low.)

See also: Annex 5, Recommendation 11, page 118.

Pain management

All women should be routinely offered pain medication (e.g. non-steroidal anti-inflammatory drugs) during both medical and surgical abortions.

General anaesthesia is not recommended routinely for vacuum aspiration abortion or dilatation and evacuation (D&E).

(Strength of recommendation: strong.
Quality of evidence based on randomized controlled trials: low.)

Remarks: Medication for pain management for both medical and surgical abortions should always be offered, and provided without delay to women who desire it. In most cases, analgesics, local anaesthesia and/or conscious sedation supplemented by verbal reassurance are sufficient, although the need for pain management increases with gestational age.

See also: Annex 5, Recommendation 14, page 118.

Recommendations for care post-abortion

Contraception

Women may start hormonal contraception at the time of surgical abortion, or as early as the time of administration of the first pill of a medical abortion regimen. Following medical abortion, an intrauterine device (IUD) may be inserted when it is reasonably certain that the woman is no longer pregnant.

(Strength of recommendation: strong.
Quality of evidence based on randomized controlled trials: very low.)

See also: Annex 5, Recommendation 13, page 118.

Follow-up

There is no medical need for a routine follow-up visit following uncomplicated surgical abortion or medical abortion using mifepristone followed by misoprostol. However, women should be advised that additional services are available to them if needed or desired.

(Strength of recommendation: strong.
Quality of the evidence based on observational studies and indirect evidence: low.)

See also: Annex 5, Recommendation 9, page 117.

Incomplete abortion

If uterine size at the time of treatment is equivalent to a pregnancy of gestational age 13 weeks or less, either vacuum aspiration or treatment with misoprostol is recommended for women with incomplete abortion. The recommended regimen of misoprostol is a single dose given either sublingually (400 μg) or orally (600 μg).

(Strength of recommendation: strong.
Quality of evidence based on randomized controlled trials: low.)

See also: Annex 5, Recommendation 10, page 117.

BOX 6

Recommendations for health systems

To the full extent of the law, safe abortion services should be readily available and affordable to all women. This means services should be available at primary-care level, with referral systems in place for all required higher-level care.

Actions to strengthen policies and services related to abortion should be based on the health needs and human rights of women and a thorough understanding of the service-delivery system and the broader social, cultural, political and economic context.

National standards and guidelines for safe abortion care should be evidence based and periodically updated, and should provide the necessary guidance to achieve equitable access to good-quality care. New policy and programme interventions should reflect evidence-based best practices. Complex service-delivery interventions require local evidence of feasibility and effectiveness through pilot-testing on a small scale prior to investing resources in scaling-up.

Training of abortion providers must ensure that they have the competencies to provide good-quality care in accordance with national standards and guidelines. Ensuring good-quality abortion care requires ongoing supervision, quality assurance, monitoring and evaluation.

Financing of abortion services should take into account costs to the health system while ensuring that services are affordable and readily available to all women who need them. Costs of adding safe abortion care to existing health services are likely to be low, relative to the costs to the health system of treating complications of unsafe abortion.

Successful scaling-up requires systematic planning, management, guidance and support for the process by which pilot interventions are both expanded and institutionalized. It also requires sufficient human and financial resources to support the process.

See Chapter 3 for further details.

BOX 7

Recommendations related to regulatory, policy and human rights considerations

Laws and policies on abortion should protect women's health and their human rights.

Regulatory, policy and programmatic barriers that hinder access to and timely provision of safe abortion care should be removed.

An enabling regulatory and policy environment is needed to ensure that every woman who is legally eligible has ready access to safe abortion care. Policies should be geared to respecting, protecting and fulfilling the human rights of women, to achieving positive health outcomes for women, to providing good-quality contraceptive information and services, and to meeting the particular needs of poor women, adolescents, rape survivors and women living with HIV.

See Chapter 4 for further details.

Process of guideline development

Background

Safe abortion: technical and policy guidance for health systems was published by the World Health Organization (WHO) in 2003 (*2*) as the first global guidance for abortion-related care and policy issues. Since that time, the guidance has been translated into French, Russian, Spanish and various non-official United Nations (UN) languages and has been widely used by governments, nongovernmental organizations (NGOs), providers of women's health services, and women's health and human rights advocates.

Since publication of the guidance in 2003, a considerable amount of new data have been produced and published, relating to epidemiological, clinical, service delivery, legal and human rights aspects of providing safe abortion care. Therefore, preparation for this revision of the guidance included extensive literature review and updating of recommendations related to service delivery, legal and policy issues, and the conduct of new systematic reviews and updates of outdated systematic reviews to provide the evidence for recommendations related to clinical questions prioritized by an international panel of experts. The substantial revisions in this update reflect changes in methods of abortion and related care, service delivery as it applies to the availability and use of new methods, and application of human rights for policy-making and legislation related to abortion, among other topics. Recommendations in the 2003 guidance for which there was no new evidence remain unchanged.

Additionally, in parallel with the revision of the guidance, a companion document entitled *Clinical practice handbook for safe abortion care* has been developed for providers of abortion services, with additional information on the details of implementing the clinical care recommendations of the guidance document.

Methods

This document was prepared according to the WHO standards and requirements for guideline development. In summary, this process included: identification of priority questions and outcomes; evidence retrieval, assessment and synthesis; formulation of recommendations; and planning for dissemination, implementation, impact evaluation and updating. The identification of priority questions for recommendations was initiated by professional staff from the WHO Department of Reproductive Health and Research (WHO Secretariat), who drafted a list of questions and outcomes related to provision of safe abortion care in light of new data since the initial publication of the guidance in 2003 (*2*), as well as in response to solicited feedback from its users.

A global panel of international stakeholders, including health-service providers, health programme managers, researchers, methodologists, human rights lawyers, and women's health and human rights advocates, was established to review and prioritize the draft questions and outcomes, which included clinical, technical and programmatic topics. This initial consultation was conducted electronically, and all responses were reviewed by members of the WHO Secretariat. Questions and outcomes rated as critical were included in the scope of this document, for evidence grading using the Grading of Recommendations Assessment, Development and Evaluation (GRADE) approach, and the development of recommendations. The list of final questions considered for GRADE tables and outcomes is presented in Annex 2.

Cochrane systematic reviews of randomized clinical trials were the primary source of evidence for the recommendations. Based on the list of priority questions, identified as described above, the relevant Cochrane systematic reviews (*3–14*) were identified and conducted or updated using their specific, standard search strategies. Additionally, three systematic reviews were conducted outside of the *Cochrane Database of Systematic Reviews* and were published in peer-reviewed journals (*15–17*). The search strategies and the specific criteria for including and excluding trials identified by the search are provided in the corresponding systematic reviews. The available evidence was appraised and graded following the GRADE approach (*18–22*), reflecting the priority comparisons and outcomes; comparisons and outcomes not relevant to the recommendation were excluded. As a result, evidence profiles (GRADE tables) were prepared (available from www.who.int/reproductivehealth/publications/unsafe_abortion/rhr_12_10). Standardized criteria for grading the evidence using GRADE are presented in Annex 3. For each selected comparison, data for available priority outcomes have been assessed and presented in the evidence profiles (if data for priority outcomes were not available in specific comparisons, they were omitted in the GRADE tables). Based on the evidence profiles, recommendations were drafted by the WHO Secretariat.

For Chapter 3 on establishing and strengthening safe abortion services, two issues were identified (indicators of safe abortion and competencies for providing safe abortion) for which recent WHO guidance was already available. Therefore, the steps taken to address the topics in Chapter 3 were to adopt and reference recent WHO guidance, and to conduct an extensive literature review of the issues presented for the existing recommendations from the first edition of the document, while updating the references.

For Chapter 4 on legal and policy considerations, WHO contracted the Programme on International Reproductive and Sexual Health Law in the Faculty of Law at the University of Toronto, Toronto, Canada, to assist the revision, including proposing changes to the existing content, based on international and regional human rights treaty provisions and the work of international and regional human rights bodies. Staff at the programme also produced a series of research briefs providing human rights and legal research and analysis on selected issues of particular concern (for example, elaboration of the health indication for safe abortion, conscientious objection, and legal and regulatory barriers).

In order to review the draft recommendations and the supporting evidence, a technical consultation was organized at WHO headquarters in Geneva, Switzerland. The members of a guidelines development group – a subset of the international panel that participated in the initial online consultation and other experts – were invited to participate in this consultation (see Annex 4 for a list of participants and their affiliations). Draft recommendations, revised chapters and supporting documents were shared with the participants before the consultation for their review.

Declarations of interest were obtained from the participants in the technical consultation using a standard WHO form prior to their participation in the meeting. These declarations were reviewed by the WHO Secretariat and, when necessary, by the WHO Office of the Legal Counsel before the consultation. Two consultation participants (Dr Laura Castleman and Dr Helena von Hertzen) declared that they were employed by organizations that have or might appear to have commercial conflicts of interest. For recommendations that were directly relevant to their organizations' work, they left the room during final recommendation making. No other participants declared any conflicts or potential conflicts of interest.

Decision-making during the technical consultation

For each recommendation, the participants in the technical consultation discussed the draft text prepared by the WHO Secretariat, with the aim of reaching consensus. Consensus was defined as agreement by the majority of participants, with no one strongly disagreeing. No strong disagreements occurred during the consultation and, therefore, an alternative system, such as voting, was not necessary. In addition to the scientific evidence and its quality, applicability issues, costs and other expert opinions were considered while formulating the final recommendations.

The strength of the recommendations was determined through the assessment of each intervention on the basis of: (i) desirable and undesirable effects; (ii) the quality of available evidence; (iii) values and preferences related to interventions in different settings; (iv) the cost of options available to health-care workers in different settings; and (v) the perceived likelihood of changing the recommendation due to further research. In general, a strong recommendation with moderate- or high-quality evidence indicates that further research should not be considered a priority. The full text of the recommendations from the technical consultation is found in Annex 5.

Topics not identified as the subject of a new systematic review for which WHO recommendations already existed were presented at the technical consultation, for group discussion. Those recommendations found by the group to be relevant and current were endorsed and adopted. These topics included: indicators of safe abortion; contraceptive use following abortion; and the recommendations surrounding establishing and strengthening abortion services, including competencies for providing abortion care, found in Chapter 3.

Document preparation and peer review

A preliminary document, containing the draft recommendations, was prepared and made available to the participants in the technical consultation three weeks before the meeting. The draft recommendations were amended during the meeting, based on the discussions. After the meeting, the draft document was revised by the WHO Secretariat. The revised version was sent electronically to all participants, for their approval and comments. Primary reviewers for each chapter were identified based on their fields of expertise. Finally, the whole document was sent for external critical appraisal and peer review. During this process of review, important suggestions were incorporated into the document; however, the WHO Secretariat refrained from making major changes in the scoping (e.g. further expansion of the guidance scoping) or in the recommendations agreed upon during the consultation.

Dissemination of the guidance document

As with the first edition of the guidance document, dissemination will be undertaken through distribution of the print version, and a series of regional workshops will be organized on applying the *WHO Strategic Approach to strengthening sexual and reproductive health policies and programmes* (23) to the issue of unsafe abortion. The aim of the workshops will be to develop proposals based on the guidance that can strengthen safe abortion care within sexual and reproductive health programmes. The workshops will include preselected country teams with representatives from ministries/departments of health, including a variety of health-service providers and programme managers, and representatives from NGOs, professional associations and UN organizations.

Assessing the impact of published guidelines is a challenging task. In an attempt to do so, we plan to monitor the number of requests from countries for assistance in implementation of the guidelines, direct follow-up in countries applying the Strategic Approach, and the number of countries that modify their national abortion programme monitoring to reflect the indicators for safe abortion provided in Table 3.2 (page 75) of this document. Additionally, we will continue to monitor the number of downloads of the document, as well as the number of hard copies of the guidance requested and distributed.

Updating the guidelines

The WHO Secretariat anticipates that these guidelines will be reviewed again four years following their publication, to assess whether revision is necessary, based upon newly available evidence and feedback from users.

References

1. *Unsafe abortion: global and regional estimates of the incidence of unsafe abortion and associated mortality in 2008*, 3rd ed. Geneva, World Health Organization, 2011.

2. *Safe abortion: technical and policy guidance for health systems.* Geneva, World Health Organization, 2003.

3. Kulier R et al. Medical methods for first trimester abortion. *Cochrane Database of Systematic Reviews*, 2004, (1):CD002855, updated 2010.

4. Kulier R et al. Surgical methods for first trimester termination of pregnancy. *Cochrane Database of Systematic Reviews*, 2001, (4):CD002900.

5. Say L et al. Medical versus surgical methods for first trimester termination of pregnancy. *Cochrane Database of Systematic Reviews*, 2005, (1):CD003037, updated 2010.

6. Lohr PA, Hayes JL, Gemzell-Danielsson K. Surgical versus medical methods for second trimester induced abortion. *Cochrane Database of Systematic Reviews*, 2008, (1):CD006714.

7. Wildschut H et al. Medical methods for mid-trimester termination of pregnancy. *Cochrane Database of Systematic Reviews*, 2011, (1):CD005216.

8. Kapp N et al. Cervical preparation for first trimester surgical abortion. *Cochrane Database of Systematic Reviews*, 2010, (2):CD007207.

9. Promsonthi P, Preechapornprasert D, Chanrachakul B. Nitric oxide donors for cervical ripening in first-trimester surgical abortion. *Cochrane Database of Systematic Reviews*, 2009, (4):CD007444.

10. Newmann SJ et al. Cervical preparation for second trimester dilation and evacuation. *Cochrane Database of Systematic Reviews*, 2010, (8):CD007310.

11. Neilson JP et al. Medical treatments for incomplete miscarriage (less than 24 weeks). *Cochrane Database of Systematic Reviews*, 2010, (1):CD007223.

12. Tunçalp O, Gülmezoglu AM, Souza JP. Surgical procedures for evacuating incomplete miscarriage. *Cochrane Database of Systematic Reviews*, 2010, (9):CD001993.

13. Mueller M et al. Antibiotic prophylaxis for medical and surgical first trimester induced abortion. *Cochrane Database of Systematic Reviews*, 2012, 2012, (3):CD005217.

14. Renner RM et al. Pain control in first trimester surgical abortion. *Cochrane Database of Systematic Reviews*, 2009, (2):CD006712.

15. Kulier R, Kapp N. Comprehensive analysis of the use of pre-procedure ultrasound for first- and second-trimester abortion. *Contraception*, 2011, 83:30–33.

16. Grossman D, Grindlay K. Alternatives to ultrasound for follow-up after medication abortion: a systematic review. *Contraception,* 2011, 83(6):504–510.

17. Jackson E, Kapp N. Pain control in first-trimester and second-trimester medical termination of pregnancy: a systematic review. *Contraception*, 2011, 83:116–126.

18. Guyatt GH et al. Incorporating considerations of resources use into grading recommendations. *British Medical Journal*, 2008, 336:1170–1173.

19. Guyatt GH et al. GRADE: an emerging consensus on rating quality of evidence and strength of recommendations. *British Medical Journal*, 336:924–926.

20. Guyatt GH et al. What is "quality of evidence" and why is it important to clinicians? *British Medical Journal*, 2008, 336:995–998.

21. Guyatt GH et al. Going from evidence to recommendations. *British Medical Journal*, 2008, 336:1049–1051.

22. Schünemann HJ et al. Grading quality of evidence and strength of recommendations for diagnostic tests and strategies. *British Medical Journal*, 2008, 336:1106–1110.

23. *The WHO Strategic Approach to strengthening sexual and reproductive health policies and programmes.* Geneva, World Health Organization, 2007.

Chapter 1

CHAPTER 1

Safe abortion care: the public health and human rights rationale

Summary

- Each year, 22 million unsafe abortions are estimated to take place. Nearly all unsafe abortions (98%) occur in developing countries. The total number of unsafe abortions has increased from about 20 million in 2003 to 22 million in 2008, although the global rate of unsafe abortion has remained unchanged since 2000.

- Approximately 47 000 pregnancy-related deaths are due to complications of unsafe abortion. In addition, 5 million women are estimated to suffer disability as a result of complications due to unsafe abortion.

- Impressive gains in contraceptive use have resulted in reducing the number of unintended pregnancies, but have not eliminated the need for access to safe abortion. An estimated 33 million contraceptive users worldwide are expected to experience accidental pregnancy annually while using contraception. Some of the accidental pregnancies are terminated by induced abortions, and some end up as unplanned births.

- Whether abortion is legally more restricted or available on request, a woman's likelihood of having an unintended pregnancy and seeking induced abortion is about the same. However, legal restrictions, together with other barriers, mean many women induce abortion themselves or seek abortion from unskilled providers. The legal status of abortion has no effect on a woman's need for an abortion, but it dramatically affects her access to safe abortion.

- Where legislation allows abortion under broad indications, the incidence of and complications from unsafe abortion are generally lower than where abortion is legally more restricted.

- In almost all countries, the law permits abortion to save the woman's life, and in the majority of countries abortion is allowed to preserve the physical and/or mental health of the woman. Therefore, safe abortion services, as provided by law, need to be available.

- Unsafe abortion and associated morbidity and mortality in women are avoidable. Safe abortion services therefore should be available and accessible for all women, to the full extent of the law.

1.1 Background

Induced abortion has been documented throughout recorded history (*1*). In earlier times, abortions were unsafe and exerted a heavy toll on women's lives. Advances in medical practice in general, and the advent of safe and effective technologies and skills to perform induced abortion in particular, could eliminate unsafe abortions and related deaths entirely, providing universal access to these services is available. Yet, an estimated 22 million abortions continue to be unsafe each year, resulting in the death of an estimated 47 000 women (*2*).

Unsafe abortion is defined by the World Health Organization (WHO) as a procedure for terminating an unintended pregnancy, carried out either by persons lacking the necessary skills or in an environment that does not conform to minimal medical standards, or both.

In nearly all developed countries (as classified by the United Nations Population Division) safe abortions are legally available upon request or under broad social and economic grounds, and services are generally accessible to most women. With the exception of a few countries, access to safe abortion in developing countries is limited to a restricted number of narrow conditions (3). In countries where abortion is legally highly restricted, unequal access to safe abortion may result. In such contexts, abortions that meet safety requirements can become the privilege of the rich, while poor women have little choice but to resort to unsafe providers, which may cause disability and death (4).

This chapter provides an overview of the health, demographic, legal and policy context of induced abortion with updated data since the publication of the document *Safe abortion: technical and policy guidance for health systems* by WHO in 2003 (5).

1.2 Public health and human rights

A consensus on the public health impact of unsafe abortion has existed for a long time. As early as 1967, the World Health Assembly identified unsafe abortion as a serious public health problem in many countries (6). WHO's *Reproductive Health Strategy to accelerate progress towards the attainment of international development goals and targets*, adopted by the World Health Assembly in 2004, noted:

"As a preventable cause of maternal mortality and morbidity, unsafe abortion must be dealt with as part of the Millennium Development Goal on improving maternal health and other international development goals and targets" (7).

The number of declarations and resolutions signed by countries over the past two decades (see for example, references 8–11) indicates a growing consensus that unsafe abortion is an important cause of maternal death that can, and should, be prevented through the promotion of sexuality education, family planning, safe abortion services to the full extent of the law, and post-abortion care in all cases. The consensus also exists that post-abortion care should always be provided, and that expanding access to modern contraception is critical to the prevention of unplanned pregnancy and unsafe abortion. Thus, the public health rationale for preventing unsafe abortion is clear and unambiguous.

Discussions that grew out of the 1968 International Conference on Human Rights in Tehran, Islamic Republic of Iran, culminated in the new concept of reproductive rights, which was subsequently defined and accepted at the 1994 International Conference on Population and Development (ICPD) in Cairo, Egypt (8). Eliminating unsafe abortion is one of the key components of the WHO *Global reproductive health strategy* (12). The strategy is grounded in international human rights treaties and global consensus declarations that call for the respect, protection and fulfilment of human rights, including the right of all persons to the highest attainable standard of health; the basic right of all couples and individuals to decide freely and responsibly the number, spacing and timing of their children and to have the information and means to do so; the right of women to have control over, and decide freely and responsibly on, matters related to their sexuality, including sexual and reproductive health – free of coercion, discrimination and violence; the right of men and women to choose a spouse and to enter into marriage only with their free and full consent; the right of access to relevant health information; and the right of every person to enjoy the benefits of scientific progress and its applications (12). To realize these rights, and to save women's lives, programmatic, legal and policy aspects of the provision of safe abortion need to be adequately addressed, as elaborated further in the following chapters.

1.3 Pregnancies and abortions

Among the 208 million women estimated to become pregnant each year worldwide, 59% (or 123 million) experience a planned (or intended) pregnancy leading to a birth or miscarriage or a stillbirth (4). The remaining 41% (or 85 million) of pregnancies are unintended.

Because of increased contraceptive use, the pregnancy rate worldwide has fallen from 160 pregnancies per 1000 women aged 15–44 years in 1995 to 134 per 1000 women in 2008 (4). Rates of intended and unintended pregnancies have fallen from, respectively, 91 and 69 per 1000 women aged 15–44 years in 1995 to 79 and 55 per 1000 women aged 15–44 years in 2008. More significantly, the rate of induced abortion has declined from 35 per 1000 women aged 15–44 years in 1995 to 26 per 1000 women aged 15–44 years in 2008. This decline has been largely due to a fall in the rate of safe abortion, while the rate of unsafe abortion has remained relatively constant since 2000 at around 14 per 1000 women aged 15–44 years (13). The absolute number of unsafe abortions was estimated at about 20 million in 2003 and 22 million in 2008. The proportion of all abortions that are unsafe has increased from 44% in 1995 and 47% in 2003 to 49% in 2008 (13). Almost all unsafe abortions occur in developing countries,

where maternal mortality rates are high and access to safe abortion is limited.

1.4 Health consequences of unsafe abortion

The health consequences of unsafe abortion depend on the facilities where abortion is performed; the skills of the abortion provider; the method of abortion used; the health of the woman; and the gestational age of her pregnancy. Unsafe abortion procedures may involve insertion of an object or substance (root, twig or catheter or traditional concoction) into the uterus; dilatation and curettage performed incorrectly by an unskilled provider; ingestion of harmful substances; and application of external force. In some settings, traditional practitioners vigorously pummel the woman's lower abdomen to disrupt the pregnancy, which can cause the uterus to rupture, killing the woman (14). The consequences of using certain medicines, such as the prostaglandin analogue misoprostol, in incorrect dosages for inducing abortion are mixed, though there is some evidence that even an incorrect dosage can still result in lowering the number of severe complications and maternal deaths (15–17).

Deaths and disability related to unsafe abortion are difficult to measure. Given that these deaths or complications occur following a clandestine or illegal procedure, stigma and fear of punishment deter reliable reporting of the incident. It is especially difficult to get reliable data on deaths from unsafe second-trimester abortions (18). Moreover, women may not relate their condition to a complication of an earlier abortion (19). Therefore, maternal deaths resulting from unsafe abortions are grossly underreported. Complications of unsafe abortion include haemorrhage, sepsis, peritonitis, and trauma to the cervix, vagina, uterus and abdominal organs (20). About 20–30% of unsafe abortions cause reproductive tract infections and 20–40% of these result in infection of the upper genital tract (21). One in four women who undergo unsafe abortion is likely to develop temporary or lifelong disability requiring medical care (22). For every woman seeking post-abortion care at a hospital, there are several who have had an unsafe abortion but who do not seek medical care, because they consider the complication as not serious, or because they may not have the required financial means, or because they fear abuse, ill-treatment or legal reprisal (23–30). Evidence shows that major physiological, financial and emotional costs are incurred by women who undergo unsafe abortion.

The burdens of unsafe abortion and of maternal deaths due to unsafe abortion are disproportionately higher for women in Africa than in any other developing region (31). For example, while Africa accounts for 27% of global births annually and for only 14% of the women aged 15–49 years in the world, its share of global unsafe abortions was 29% and, more seriously, 62% of all deaths related to unsafe abortion occurred in Africa in 2008 (see Figure 1.1). The risk of death due to unsafe abortion varies among developing regions. The case–fatality rate for unsafe abortion is 460 per 100 000 unsafe abortion procedures in Africa and 520 per 100 000 in sub-Saharan Africa, compared with 30 per 100 000 in Latin America and the Caribbean and 160 per 100 000 in Asia (2).

Figure 1.1 The percentage distribution of women, births, unsafe abortions and related deaths, by developing region, 2008

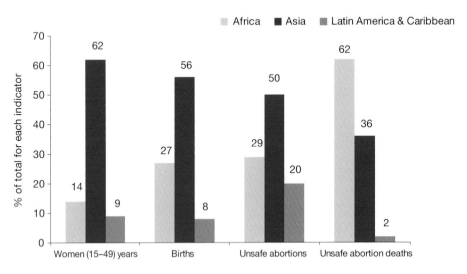

Reproduced from reference 31.

Safe abortion care: the public health and human rights rationale

When performed by skilled providers using correct medical techniques and drugs, and under hygienic conditions, induced abortion is a very safe medical procedure. In the United States of America (USA), for example, the case–fatality rate is 0.7 per 100 000 legal abortions (32). Late second-trimester legal abortion has a case–fatality rate (33) that is much lower than the lowest rate of unsafe abortion procedures (see Figures 1.2 and 1.3).

Figure 1.2 Case–fatality rates of legal induced abortions, spontaneous abortions or term deliveries, per 100 000 procedures, USA   Reproduced, with permission, from reference *32*.

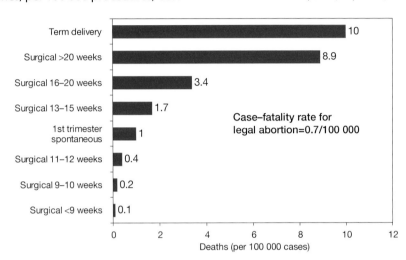

Figure 1.3 Case–fatality rates per 100 000 unsafe abortion procedures, by region, 2008   Reproduced from reference *2*.

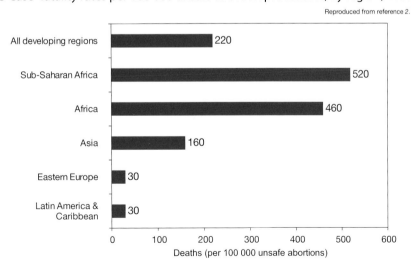

1.5 Contraceptive use, accidental pregnancies and unmet need for family planning

The prevalence of contraception of any method was 63% globally in 2007 among women of reproductive age (15–49 years) who were married or in a cohabiting union (*34*). The use of a modern method was about seven percentage points lower, at 56%. Contraceptive prevalence rose globally and in all regions, though it remains low in Africa, at 28% for all methods and 22% for modern methods (see Figure 1.4). The prevalence is even lower in sub-Saharan Africa, where, in 2007, the use of any contraceptive method was 21%, while the use of modern methods was 15%. In contrast, contraceptive prevalence of any method was over 66% in Europe, North America, Asia, and Latin America and the Caribbean.

The use of modern contraception has resulted in a lowering of the incidence and prevalence of induced abortion even where abortion is available on request. The decline in abortion prevalence with the increase in the level of contraceptive prevalence has been examined by several authors (*35, 36*). Recent data from 12 countries in eastern Europe and central Asia, where induced abortion used to be the main method for regulating fertility, and from the USA, show that where the use of modern contraceptive methods is high, the incidence of induced abortion is low (*37*). Rates of induced abortion are the lowest in western Europe, where modern contraceptive use is high and abortion is generally legally available on request. Meeting the unmet need for family planning is, therefore, an effective intervention to reduce unintended pregnancy and induced abortion.

Contraception alone, however, cannot entirely eliminate women's need for access to safe abortion services. Contraception plays no role in cases of forced sexual intercourse, which can lead to an unintended pregnancy. Also, no method is 100% effective in

Figure 1.4 Percentage of women who are married or in cohabiting union, using any method or modern method of contraception, 2007

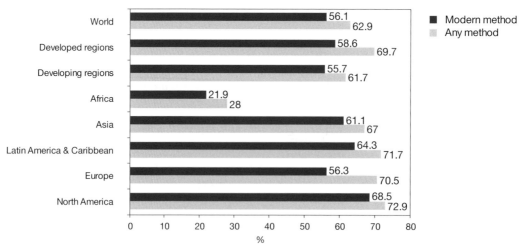

Reproduced from reference *34*.

preventing pregnancy. Using 2007 data on contraceptive prevalence (*34*) and the typical failure rates of contraceptive methods (*51*), it is estimated that approximately 33 million women worldwide annually may experience an accidental pregnancy while using a method of contraception (see Table 1.1). In the absence of safe abortion services, some may resort to unskilled providers and the others may end up having unwanted births. The implications of unwanted births are not well studied, but the effects can be harmful and long-lasting for women and for those who are born unwanted (*38*).

Unmet need for family planning, broadly defined as the number of women who want to avoid or postpone a pregnancy but are not using any method of contraception, continues to persist, despite having declined somewhat (*39*). Overall, 11% of women in developing countries report an unmet need for family planning. In sub-Saharan Africa and among the least developed countries, unmet need for family planning is reported by one in four women in the reproductive age group of 15–49 years (*39*). Women will continue to face unintended pregnancies as long as their family planning needs are not met.

Unlike unmet need for family planning, the lack of access to safe abortion care is less well documented, except for the stark reality of an estimated 22 million women undergoing unsafe abortion each year (*2*), with 47 000 of them dying from the complications. Even a "low-risk" unsafe abortion in a legally restricted context exposes women to an undue risk should an emergency develop in the process. In such cases, because of legal restrictions and stigma linked to having an abortion, women may be reluctant to seek timely medical care if post-abortion complications occur.

1.6 Regulatory and policy context

Where laws and policies allow abortion under broad indications, the incidence of, and mortality from, unsafe abortion are reduced to a minimum (*2*). Abortion is permitted for social or economic reasons in only 16% of developing countries as compared with 80% of developed countries (see Table 1.2). Three out of four induced abortions in developing countries (excluding the People's Republic of China) are carried out in unsafe conditions (*13*). In these countries, few women meet the legal conditions, or know their right, to receive the safe abortion services to which they are legally entitled. Also, providers may not be aware of the legal provisions or may be unwilling to provide legal abortion services. Furthermore, in some countries, laws are not applied (*40*).

Whether abortion is legally restricted or not, the likelihood that a woman will have an abortion for an unintended pregnancy is about the same (*13*). The legal restrictions lead many women to seek services in other countries, or from unskilled providers or under unhygienic conditions, exposing them to a significant risk of death or disability. The maternal mortality ratio per 100 000 live births due to unsafe abortion is generally higher in countries with major restrictions and lower in countries where abortion is available on request or under broad conditions (*41, 42*). The accumulated evidence shows that the removal of restrictions on abortion results in reduction of maternal mortality due to unsafe abortion and, thus, a reduction in the overall level of maternal mortality (*43, 44, 45, 46*).

In a small number of countries, where maternal mortality is low despite restrictive abortion laws, many women have access to safe or relatively safe abortion through seeking care from neighbouring countries, through provision of safe, but illegal abortion care domestically, or through self-use of misoprostol (*47–49*).

In addition to the legal restrictions, other barriers to safe abortion include inability to pay, lack of social support, delays in seeking health-care, providers' negative attitudes, and poor quality of services. Young women are especially vulnerable where effective contraceptive methods are available only to married women or where the incidence of non-consensual sexual intercourse is high. Nearly 14% of all unsafe abortions in developing countries are among women aged under 20 years. In Africa, young women below the age of 25 years account for nearly two thirds of all unsafe abortions in that region (50). A higher percentage of young women, compared with adult women, tend to have second-trimester abortions, which are more risky.

Table 1.1 Estimated number of women using a contraceptive method and those experiencing an unintended pregnancy during the first year of contraceptive use, by type of contraceptive method, global data, 2007

Contraceptive method	Estimated failure rate (typical use), %[a]	Number of users, thousands[b]	Number of women with accidental pregnancy (typical use), thousands[c]
Female sterilization	0.5	232 564	1163
Male sterilization	0.15	32 078	48
Injectables	0.3	42 389	127
Intrauterine device (IUD)	0.8	162 680	1301
Pill	5.0	100 816	5041
Male condom	14	69 884	9784
Vaginal barrier	20	2291	458
Periodic abstinence	25	37 806	9452
Withdrawal	19	32 078	6095
Total	4.7	712 586	33 469

[a] Trussell (51) estimates are based on USA data. Estimated failure rates in typical use cover method failure and user failure in using a contraceptive method in typical conditions.

[b] Based on the estimated number of women aged 15–49 years, married or in union in 2007 and the percentage using a specific contraceptive method (34).

[c] Column (4) = Column(3) × (Column(2)/100)

Safe abortion care: the public health and human rights rationale

Table 1.2 Grounds on which abortion is permitted (% of countries) by region and subregion, 2009

Country or area	To save the woman's life	To preserve physical health	To preserve mental health	Rape or incest	Fetal impairment	Economic or social reasons	On request	Number of countries
All countries	97	67	63	49	47	34	29	195
Developed countries	96	88	86	84	84	80	69	49
Developing countries	97	60	55	37	34	19	16	146
Africa	100	60	55	32	32	8	6	53
Eastern Africa	100	71	65	18	24	6	0	17
Middle Africa	100	33	22	11	11	0	0	9
Northern Africa	100	50	50	33	17	17	17	6
Southern Africa	100	80	80	60	80	20	20	5
Western Africa	100	63	56	50	44	6	6	16
Asia[a]	100	63	61	50	54	39	37	46
Eastern Asia	100	100	100	100	100	75	75	4
South-central Asia	100	64	64	57	50	50	43	14
South-eastern Asia	100	55	45	36	36	27	27	11
Western Asia	100	59	59	41	59	29	29	17
Latin America and the Caribbean	88	58	52	36	21	18	9	33
Caribbean	92	69	69	38	23	23	8	13
Central America	75	50	38	25	25	25	13	8
South America	92	50	42	42	17	8	8	12
Oceania[a]	100	50	50	14	7	0	0	14

[a] Japan, Australia and New Zealand have been excluded from the regional count, but are included in the total for developed countries.

Adapted from reference 3.

1.7 Economic costs of unsafe abortion

Safe abortion is cost saving. The cost to health systems of treating the complications of unsafe abortion is overwhelming, especially in poor countries. The overall average cost per case that governments incur is estimated (in 2006 US dollars) at US$ 114 for Africa and US$ 130 for Latin America (52). The economic costs of unsafe abortion to a country's health system, however, go beyond the direct costs of providing post-abortion services. A recent study (52) estimated an annual cost of US$ 23 million for treating minor complications from unsafe abortion at the primary health-care level; US$ 6 billion for treating post-abortion infertility; and US$ 200 million each year for the out-of-pocket expenses of individuals and households in sub-Saharan Africa for the treatment of post-abortion complications. In addition, US$ 930 million is the estimated annual expenditure by individuals and their societies for lost income from death or long-term disability due to chronic health consequences of unsafe abortion (52).

Unsafe abortion was estimated to cost the Mexico City health system US$ 2.6 million in 2005, before the legalization of abortion (53). With access to safe abortion, the system could potentially save US$ 1.7 million annually. A large amount of money can thus be conserved and redirected to meeting other urgent needs, including the provision of quality services using up-to-date standards and guidelines, trained providers and appropriate technologies, if unintended pregnancies are prevented by effective contraception, and safe abortion is accessible. Economic grounds further strengthen the public-health and human-rights rationale for the provision of safe abortion.

Safe abortion care: the public health and human rights rationale

References

1. Joffe C. Abortion and medicine: a sociopolitical history. In Paul M et al., eds. *Management of unintended and abnormal pregnancy: comprehensive abortion care.* Oxford, Wiley-Blackwell, 2009:1–9.

2. *Unsafe abortion: global and regional estimates of the incidence of unsafe abortion and associated mortality in 2008*, 6th ed. Geneva, World Health Organization, 2011.

3. United Nations, Department for Economic and Social Affairs, Population Division. *World abortion policies*. New York, United Nations, 2011 (ST/ESA/SER.A/302).

4. Singh S et al. *Abortion worldwide: a decade of uneven progress*. New York, Guttmacher Institute, 2009.

5. *Safe abortion: technical and policy guidance for health systems.* Geneva, World Health Organization, 2003.

6. Resolution WHA20.41. Health aspects of population dynamics. In: *Twentieth World Health Assembly, Geneva, 23 May 1967.* Geneva, World Health Organization, 1967 (WHA20/1967/REC/1).

7. Resolution WHA57.12. Reproductive health: strategy to accelerate progress towards the attainment of international development goals and targets. In: *Fifty-seventh World Health Assembly, Geneva, 17–22 May 2004.* Geneva, World Health Organization, 2004 (WHA57/2004/REC/1).

8. *International Conference on Population and Development – ICPD – Programme of Action.* New York, United Nations Population Fund, 1995 (A/CONF171/13/Rev.1 (http://www.unfpa.org/webdav/site/global/shared/documents/publications/2004/icpd_eng.pdf, accessed 31 August 2011).

9. Resolution S-21.2. Key actions for the further implementation of the Programme of Action of the International Conference on Population and development. In: *Twenty-first special session of the United Nations General Assembly New York, 30 June–2 July 1999.* New York, United Nations, 1999 (A/RES/S-21/2).

10. *Plan of action on sexual and reproductive health and rights (Maputo Plan of Action).* Addis Ababa, The African Union Commission, 2006 (http://www.unfpa.org/africa/newdocs/maputo_eng.pdf, accessed 31 August 2011).

11. *Access to safe and legal abortion in Europe.* Strasbourg, Council of Europe, 2008 (Resolution 1607 of the Parliamentary Assembly of the Council of Europe; http://assembly.coe.int/Main.asp?link=/Documents/AdoptedText/ta08/ERES1607.htm, accessed 31 August 2011).

12. *Reproductive health strategy to accelerate progress towards the attainment of international development goals and targets.* Geneva, World Health Organization, 2004.

13. Sedgh G, et al. Induced abortion: incidence and trends worldwide from 1995 to 2008. *Lancet,* 2012, 379:625–632.

14. Ugboma HA, Akani CI. Abdominal massage: another cause of maternal mortality. *Nigerian Journal of Medicine*, 2004, 13:259–262.

15. Harper CC et al. Reducing maternal mortality due to elective abortion: potential impact of misoprostol in low-resource settings. *International Journal of Gynecology and Obstetrics*, 2007, 98:66–69.

16. Miller S et al. Misoprostol and declining abortion-related morbidity in Santo Domingo, Dominican Republic: a temporal association. *British Journal of Obstetrics and Gynaecology*, 2005, 112:1291–1296.

17. Sherris J et al. Misoprostol use in developing countries: results from a multicountry study. *International Journal of Obstetrics and Gynecology*, 2005, 88:76–81.

18. Walker D et al. Deaths from complications of unsafe abortion: misclassified second trimester deaths. *Reproductive Health Matters*, 2004, 12:27–38.

19. Benson J. Evaluating abortion-care programs: old challenges, new directions. *Studies in Family Planning*, 2005, 36:189–202.

20. Grimes D et al. Unsafe abortion: the preventable pandemic. *Lancet*, 2006, 368:1908–1919.

21. *Unsafe abortion: global and regional estimates of incidence of unsafe abortion and associated mortality in 2000*, 4th ed. Geneva, World Health Organization, 2004.

22. Singh S. Hospital admissions resulting from unsafe abortion: estimates from 13 developing countries. *Lancet*, 2006, 368:1887–1892.

23. Singh S, Wulf D. Estimated levels of induced abortion in six Latin American countries. *International Family Planning Perspectives*, 1994, 20:4–13.

24. Singh S, Wulf D, Jones H. Health professionals' perceptions about induced abortion in South Central and Southeast Asia. *International Family Planning Perspectives*, 1997, 23:59–67 and 72.

25. Singh S et al. Estimating the level of abortion in the Philippines and Bangladesh. *International Family Planning Perspectives*, 1997, 23:100–107 and 144.

26. Juarez F et al. Incidence of induced abortions in the Philippines: current level and trends. *International Family Planning Perspectives*, 2005, 31:140–149.

27. Singh S et al. The incidence of induced abortion in Uganda. *International Family Planning Perspectives*, 2005, 31:183–191.

28. Huntington D. Abortion in Egypt: official constraints and popular practices. In: Makhlouf Obermeyer C, ed. *Cross-cultural perspectives on reproductive health.* New York, Oxford University Press, 2001:175–192.

29. Ferrando D. *El aborto inducido en el Peru, hechos y cifras.* [Clandestine abortion in Peru, facts and figures.] Lima, Centro de la Mujer Peruana Flora Tristán and Pathfinder International, 2002.

30. *Unwanted pregnancy and postabortion complications in Pakistan. Findings from a national study.* Islamabad, The Population Council, 2002.

31. Shah I, Ahman E. Unsafe abortion: global and regional incidence, trends, consequences and challenges. *Journal of Obstetrics and Gynaecology Canada*, 2009, 1149–1158.

32. Bartlett LA et al. Risk factors for legal induced abortion-related mortality in the United States. *Obstetrics and Gynecology*, 2004, 103:729–737.

33. Lichtenberg E, Grimes D. Surgical complications: prevention and management. In Paul M et al., eds. *Management of unintended and abnormal pregnancy: comprehensive abortion care.* Oxford, Wiley-Blackwell, 2009:224–251.

34. United Nations, Department for Economic and Social Affairs, Population Division. *World contraceptive use (wallchart).* New York, United Nations, 2009 (ST/ESA/SER.A/285).

35. Bongaarts J, Westoff C. The potential role of contraception in reducing abortion. *Studies in Family Planning*, 2000, 31:193–202.

36. Marston C, Cleland J. Relationships between contraception and abortion: a review of the evidence. *International Family Planning Perspectives*, 2003, 29:6–13.

37. Westoff CF. *Recent trends in abortion and contraception in 12 countries.* Washington, DC, ORC Macro, 2005, No. 8.

38. David HP. Born unwanted, 35 years later: the Prague study. *Reproductive Health Matters*, 2006, 14:181–190.

39. *The Millennium Development Goals report 2010: statistical annexes.* New York, United Nations, 2010.

40. Schuster S. Women's experiences of the abortion law in Cameroon: "What really matters". *Reproductive Health Matters*, 2010, 18:137–144.

41. *World Health Report 2008 – primary health care: now more than ever.* Geneva, World Health Organization, 2008.

42. *Women and health: today's evidence, tomorrow's agenda.* Geneva, World Health Organization, 2009.

43. David HP. Abortion in Europe, 1920–91 – a public-health perspective. *Studies in Family Planning*, 1992, 23:1–22.

44. Jewkes R et al. Prevalence of morbidity associated with abortion before and after legalisation in South Africa. *British Medical Journal*, 2002, 324:1252–1253.

45. Jewkes R and Rees H, Dramatic decline in abortion mortality due to the Choice on Termination of Pregnancy Act. *South African Medical Journal*, 2005, 95[4]:250.

46. Pradhan A et al., Nepal Maternal Mortality and Morbidity Study 2008/2009: Summary of Preliminary Findings, Kathmandu, Nepal: Family Health Division, Department of Health Services, Ministry of Health, 2009.

47. Kulczycki A. Abortion in Latin America: changes in practice, growing conflict, and recent policy developments. *Studies in Family Planning*, 2011, 42(3):199–220.

48. Briozzo L et al. A risk reduction strategy to prevent maternal deaths associated with unsafe abortion. *International Journal of Gynecology and Obstetrics,* 2006, 95(2):221–226.

49. Payne D. More British abortions for Irish women. *British Medical Journal,* 1999, 318(7176):77.

50. *Unsafe abortion: global and regional estimates of the incidence of unsafe abortion and associated mortality in 2003*, 5th ed. Geneva, World Health Organization, 2007.

51. Trussell J. Contraceptive efficacy. In: Hatcher RA, et al. eds. *Contraceptive technology*, 17th revised ed. New York, Ardent Media, 1998:779–884. Levin C et al. Exploring the costs and economic consequences of unsafe abortion in Mexico City before legalisation. *Reproductive Health Matters*, 2009, 17:120–132.

52. Vlassoff M et al. *Economic impact of unsafe abortion-related morbidity and mortality: evidence and estimation challenges*. Brighton, Institute of Development Studies, 2008 (IDS Research Reports 59).

53. Levin C et al. Exploring the costs and economic consequences of unsafe abortion in Mexico City before legalisation. *Reproductive Health Matters*, 2009, 17:120–132.

Chapter 2

CHAPTER 2
Clinical care for women undergoing abortion

Summary

This chapter addresses, in brief, the clinical management of women before, during and after their abortion. Providing clinical care for women undergoing abortion is described in greater detail in the WHO document *Clinical practice handbook for safe abortion care*.

The evidence base for the following recommendations are available as GRADE (Grading of Recommendations Assessment, Development and Evaluation) tables and accessible online. Details of the GRADE methodology are presented in the Methods section of this document (pages 10–11). GRADE tables are available from: www.who.int/reproductivehealth/publications/unsafe_abortion/rhr_12_10.

Pre-abortion care

- Determining the gestational age is a critical factor in selecting the most appropriate abortion method. Bimanual pelvic examination, abdominal examination and recognition of symptoms of pregnancy are usually adequate. Laboratory or ultrasound testing may also be used, if needed.

- Routine use of antibiotics at the time of surgical abortion reduces the post-procedural risk of infection. However, abortion should not be denied when prophylactic antibiotics are not available (GRADE tables 66–70).

- Complete, accurate and easy-to-understand information about the procedure and what to expect during and afterwards must be given to the woman in a format that is accessible to her and helps with her decision-making and voluntary consent. Information regarding post-abortion contraception also needs to be provided.

Methods of abortion

- The following methods are recommended for first-trimester abortion:

  - manual or electric vacuum aspiration, for pregnancies of gestational age up to 12–14 weeks (GRADE tables 36 and 37);

  - medical method of abortion, specifically, oral mifepristone followed by a single dose of misoprostol, for pregnancies of gestational age up to 9 weeks (63 days) (GRADE tables 30–32);

  - medical method of abortion for pregnancies of gestational age over 9 weeks (63 days) – oral mifepristone followed by repeated doses of misoprostol (GRADE tables 94–121); or

  - where mifepristone is not available: misoprostol alone, in repeated doses (GRADE table 113).

- Dilatation and curettage (D&C) is an obsolete method of surgical abortion and should be replaced by vacuum aspiration and/or medical methods (GRADE table 35).

- For pregnancies of gestational age more than 12–14 weeks, the following methods are recommended:

- dilatation and evacuation (D&E), using vacuum aspiration and forceps (GRADE tables 33 and 34); or

- mifepristone followed by repeated doses of misoprostol (GRADE tables 71–92); or

- where mifepristone is not available, misoprostol alone, in repeated doses (GRADE tables 71–92).

- Cervical preparation before surgical abortion is recommended for all women with a pregnancy of gestational age over 12–14 weeks, although its use may be considered for women at any gestational age, in particular those at high risk for cervical injury or uterine perforation (GRADE tables 1–19).

- Medication for pain management for both medical and surgical abortions should always be offered, and provided without delay to women who desire it (GRADE tables 38–60, 125–132). In most cases, analgesics, local anaesthesia and/or conscious sedation supplemented by verbal reassurance are sufficient. The need for pain management increases with gestational age.

- Local anaesthesia, such as lidocaine, can be used to alleviate women's discomfort where mechanical cervical dilatation is required for surgical abortion. General anaesthesia is not recommended for routine abortion procedures, as it has been associated with higher rates of complications than analgesia and local anaesthesia (GRADE tables 38–60).

- Standard precautions for infection control should be used, as with the care of all patients at all times, to reduce the risk of transmission of bloodborne infections (http://www.who.int/csr/resources/publications/EPR_AM2_E7.pdf).

After-care and follow-up

- For surgical abortion, women can leave the health-care facility as soon as they feel able and their vital signs are normal.

- Following uncomplicated surgical and medical abortion using mifepristone with misoprostol, routine follow-up visits are not necessary. For women who wish to return to the clinic, a follow-up visit may be scheduled at 7–14 days after the procedure (GRADE table 93).

- Before leaving the health-care facility following the surgical abortion procedure or administration of medical abortion pills, all women should receive contraceptive information and, if desired, the contraceptive method of their choice or referral for such services (http://www.who.int/reproductivehealth/publications/family_planning/9789241563888/en/index.html).

- Before leaving the facility women should receive oral and written instructions about how to care for themselves after they leave. These instructions should include: how much bleeding to expect, how to recognize potential complications, and how and where to seek help if required. Where possible, a phone number that women could call to ask questions or express concerns may reduce the need to return to the clinic.

2.1 Pre-abortion care

The first steps in providing abortion care are to establish that the woman is indeed pregnant and, if so, to estimate the duration of the pregnancy and confirm that the pregnancy is intrauterine. The risks associated with induced abortion, though small when abortion is properly performed, increase with the duration of pregnancy (1, 2). Determination of the length of pregnancy is a critical factor in selecting the most appropriate abortion method, and determines the content of the information and counselling to be given to women prior to abortion. Every health-service-delivery point should have staff who are trained and competent to take the woman's medical history and perform a bimanual pelvic and an abdominal examination to accurately assess pregnancy and its duration. Health-care centres that are not staffed and equipped to provide induced abortion must be able to refer women promptly to the nearest services with minimal delay. Staff should also be competent to offer counselling to help the woman consider her options if needed (see Section 2.1.8).

2.1.1 Medical history

Most women begin to suspect that they are pregnant when their expected menstrual period does not occur. The woman should be asked about the first day of her last menstrual period (LMP), i.e. the first day of bleeding and whether the menstruation was normal, as well as about her menstrual history, including the regularity of her cycles. Women may experience amenorrhoea for reasons other than pregnancy, however, and some women who are pregnant may not report having missed a period. For example, women who are breastfeeding may become pregnant before their first postpartum menses, and women who are amenorrhoeic while using injectable hormonal contraception may become pregnant after missing an injection. Some women may experience non-menstrual bleeding in early pregnancy, and this can be a cause of missing or misdating pregnancy. Other symptoms that women commonly report in early pregnancy include breast tenderness and engorgement, nausea sometimes accompanied by vomiting, fatigue, changes in appetite, and increased frequency of urination.

In addition to estimating the duration of pregnancy, clinical history-taking should serve to identify

contraindications to medical or surgical abortion methods and to identify risk factors for complications of treatment. History-taking should include: personal and family history of relevant diseases; obstetric and gynaecologic history, including previous ectopic pregnancy; any bleeding tendencies or disorders; history of or presence of sexually transmitted infections (STIs); current use of medications; known allergies; and risk assessment for violence or coercion. The health-care provider must be alert to the possibility of violence or coercion in the context of unintended pregnancy (see Section 2.1.8.1).

From a clinical point of view, the presence of HIV infection in a woman undergoing abortion requires the same precautions as for other medical/surgical interventions (see Section 2.2.7.1). HIV testing may be offered but is not required for women to receive induced abortion services.

2.1.2 Physical examination

Basic routine observations (pulse, blood pressure and, in some cases, temperature) are useful baseline measurements. Additionally, health-care providers must confirm pregnancy and estimate its duration by a bimanual pelvic and an abdominal examination. While many health-care workers have been trained to assess the length of pregnancy in order to provide prenatal care, many are not experienced in diagnosing very early pregnancy or accurately estimating the duration of pregnancy during the first trimester. Hence, additional training in bimanual pelvic examination is often required for staff who intend to provide abortion services (see Chapter 3).

Signs of pregnancy that are detectable during a bimanual pelvic examination as early as 6–8 weeks of gestation include softening of the cervical isthmus and softening and enlargement of the uterus. A pregnant woman's uterus that is smaller than expected could be due to a pregnancy that is less advanced than estimated from the date of the LMP, an ectopic pregnancy, or a missed abortion; a uterus that is larger than expected may indicate a pregnancy that is more advanced than calculated from the date of the LMP, a multiple pregnancy, a full bladder, the presence of uterine fibroids or other pelvic tumours, or a molar pregnancy. A physical examination is generally more accurate and reliable if the woman empties her bladder prior to the examination.

During the physical examination, the health-care provider should also assess whether the uterus is anteverted, retroverted or otherwise positioned in a way that might affect assessment of the gestational age or complicate a surgical abortion. Health-care providers should be trained to recognize signs of STIs and other reproductive tract infections (RTIs), as well as health conditions, such as anaemia or malaria, that may require additional procedures or services, or referral.

2.1.3 Laboratory testing

In most cases, health-care providers only require the information obtained from the woman's history and from a physical examination to confirm the pregnancy and estimate its duration. Laboratory testing for pregnancy is not needed, unless the typical signs of pregnancy are not clearly present and the provider is unsure whether the woman is pregnant. Obtaining such tests should not hinder or delay uterine evacuation.

Routine laboratory testing is not a prerequisite for abortion services. Measuring haemoglobin or haematocrit levels to detect anaemia may be useful when initiating treatment in the rare cases of haemorrhage occurring at the time of or following the abortion procedure. Tests for Rhesus (Rh) blood group typing should be provided when feasible, to

administer Rh-immunoglobulin when indicated (see Section 2.1.7).

2.1.4 Ultrasound scanning

Ultrasound scanning is not routinely required for the provision of abortion (3–5) (GRADE tables 122–124). Where it is available, a scan can help identify an intrauterine pregnancy and exclude an ectopic one from 6 weeks of gestation (6). It may also help determine gestational age and diagnose pathologies or non-viability of a pregnancy. Some health-care providers find the technology helpful before or during D&E. Where ultrasound is used, service-delivery sites should, if possible, provide separate areas where women seeking abortion can be scanned, away from those receiving prenatal/antenatal care.

2.1.5 Reproductive tract infections

The presence of infection in the lower reproductive tract at the time of abortion is a risk factor for post-surgical abortion RTIs (7). The routine use of antibiotics at the time of surgical abortion has been reported to reduce the post-procedural risk of infection by half (8, 9). However, where antibiotics are not available for prophylactic use, abortion may still be performed. In all cases, strict observation of cleaning and disinfection procedures should be followed (see Section 2.2.7.1).

Following medical abortion, the risk of intrauterine infection is very low and prophylactic antibiotics are therefore not necessary (10) (GRADE table 70).

If clinical signs indicate infection, the woman should be treated immediately with antibiotics, and abortion can then be performed. Where laboratory testing for STIs is routinely performed, and if there are no visible signs of infection, abortion should not be delayed to wait for the test results.

2.1.6 Ectopic pregnancy

Ectopic pregnancy is an uncommon, but potentially life-threatening event, occurring in 1.5–2% of pregnancies. Signs and symptoms that might indicate extrauterine pregnancy include uterine size smaller than expected for the estimated length of pregnancy; cervical motion tenderness, lower abdominal pain, especially if accompanied by vaginal bleeding and spotting; dizziness or fainting; pallor; and, in some women, an adnexal mass. If ectopic pregnancy is suspected, it is essential to confirm the diagnosis immediately and to initiate treatment or transfer the woman as soon as possible to a facility that has the capacity to confirm diagnosis and provide treatment (11). The inspection of aspirated tissue following a surgical abortion procedure can nearly eliminate the risk of an ectopic pregnancy going undetected (see Section 2.2.4.5).

It should be noted that it is more difficult to diagnose an ectopic pregnancy during and after medical methods of abortion, due to the similarity of symptoms (12). Additionally, neither mifepristone nor misoprostol are treatments for ectopic pregnancy, which, if present, will continue to grow. Therefore, health-care staff must be particularly alert to clinical signs of ectopic pregnancy, such as a uterus that feels smaller than expected according to the date of the woman's LMP, cervical motion tenderness, or the presence of an adnexal mass on pelvic examination (13). Women should be told to seek medical advice promptly if they experience symptoms that may indicate ectopic pregnancy, such as severe and intensifying abdominal pain, particularly if it is one-sided.

Where clinical features (e.g. history of previous ectopic pregnancy or pelvic inflammatory disease, discrepancy between menstrual dates and assessment of gestational age, vaginal bleeding, pregnancy in the presence of an intrauterine device (IUD), or pelvic pain) raise suspicion of an ectopic pregnancy, further investigations should be performed (14). These may include pelvic ultrasound and serial human chorionic gonadotrophin (hCG) measurements. If these are not possible, or if ectopic pregnancy is diagnosed or strongly suspected, the woman should be transferred to an appropriate referral centre for treatment.

2.1.7 Rh-isoimmunization

Passive immunization of all Rh-negative women with Rh-immunoglobulin within 72 hours after abortion was recommended in the USA in 1961 (15), yet there is still no conclusive evidence about the need for this measure after early induced abortion (16). In settings where the prevalence of Rh-negative status is high, and Rh-immunoglobulin is routinely provided in the facility to Rh-negative women, it should be administered at the time of the abortion procedure. The dose of Rh-immunoglobulin may be reduced from 300 µg (the dose given after term delivery) to 50 µg in pregnancies of less than 12 weeks' duration (17). Rh testing is not a requirement for abortion services where it is not available or the prevalence of Rh-negative status is low.

In pregnancies up to 9 weeks' (63 days') gestation, however, the theoretical risk of maternal Rh-sensitization with medical abortion is very low (17). Thus, determination of Rh status and the offer of anti-D prophylaxis are not considered prerequisites for early medical abortion (12). If Rh-immunoglobulin is available, administration of the immunoglobulin to Rh-negative women having a medical abortion is recommended at the time of the prostaglandin administration (18). For women using misoprostol at home, Rh-immunoglobulin may be administered at the time mifepristone is taken.

2.1.8 Information and counselling

The provision of information is an essential part of good-quality abortion services (*19*). Every pregnant woman who is contemplating abortion should receive adequate relevant information and be offered counselling from a trained health-care professional with comprehensive knowledge and experience of different methods of abortion. Information must be provided to each woman, regardless of her age or circumstances, in a way that she can understand, to allow her to make her own decisions about whether to have an abortion and, if so, what method to choose.

Information, counselling and abortion procedures should be provided as promptly as possible without undue delay. Chapter 3 presents details about training and other health-care provider requirements related to the provision of information and counselling, including ethical standards.

2.1.8.1 Decision-making information and counselling

Providing information and offering counselling can be very important in helping the woman consider her options and ensuring that she can make a decision that is free from pressure. Many women have made a decision to have an abortion before seeking care, and this decision should be respected without subjecting a woman to mandatory counselling. Provision of counselling to women who desire it should be voluntary, confidential, non-directive and by a trained person (*19, 20*).

If the woman chooses an abortion, the health-care worker should explain any legal requirements for obtaining it. The woman should be given as much time as she needs to make her decision, even if it means returning to the clinic later. However, the advantage of abortion at earlier gestational ages in terms of their greater safety over abortion at later ages should be explained. Once the decision is made by the woman, abortion should be provided as soon as is possible to do so (*19*). The health-care worker should also provide information and referral for antenatal care to women who decide to carry the pregnancy to term and/or consider adoption.

In some circumstances, the woman may be under pressure from her partner, family members, health-care providers or others to have an abortion. Unmarried adolescents, women in abusive relationships and women living with HIV may be particularly vulnerable to such pressure. If health-care workers suspect coercion, they should talk with the woman alone, or refer her for additional counselling. If staff know or suspect that the woman has been subjected to sexual violence or other abuse, they should offer her referrals for other counselling and treatment services as appropriate. Managers should ensure that all staff know about the availability of such resources in the health system and the community (see Chapter 3).

2.1.8.2 Information on abortion procedures

At a minimum, a woman must be given information on:

- what will be done during and after the procedure;

- what she is likely to experience (e.g. menstrual-like cramps, pain and bleeding);

- how long the process is likely to take;

- what pain management will be made available to her;

- risks and complications associated with the abortion method;

- when she will be able to resume her normal activities, including sexual intercourse;

- any follow-up care.

If a choice of abortion methods is available, health-care providers should be trained to give women clear information about which methods are appropriate, based on the duration of pregnancy and the woman's medical condition, as well as potential risk factors and the advantages and disadvantages of each available method. Women are more likely to find a method of abortion acceptable if they have chosen it themselves (21, 22). Having a choice of methods is seen as extremely important by the majority of women undergoing abortion. Several studies suggest, however, that women who choose medical abortion find it more acceptable at earlier gestations when compared with later gestations (21, 23–25).

2.1.8.3 Contraceptive information and services

The goal of contraceptive counselling and provision in the context of abortion care is to begin the chosen method immediately following abortion, after ensuring that it is the most appropriate and acceptable method for the woman. This will increase the likelihood that she will continue its correct and consistent use. Provision of contraceptive information, and offers of counselling, methods and services is an essential part of abortion care, as it helps the woman avoid unintended pregnancies in the future. Ideally, pre-abortion counselling includes discussion about future contraceptive needs. Every woman should be informed that ovulation can return as early as 2 weeks after abortion (26), putting her at risk of pregnancy unless an effective contraceptive method is used. She should be given accurate information to assist her in choosing the most appropriate contraceptive method to meet her needs. In helping the woman choose the most appropriate contraceptive method for the future, it may be useful to explore the circumstances in which the unintended pregnancy occurred. If the woman is seeking an abortion following what she considers to be a contraceptive failure,

the health-care provider should discuss whether the method may have been used incorrectly and how to use it correctly, or whether it may be appropriate for her to change to a different method (for further discussion, see Section 2.3 and Annex 6). The final selection of a method, however, must be the woman's alone.

A woman's acceptance of a contraceptive method must never be a precondition for providing her an abortion. Some women may prefer to discuss options for contraception after their abortion is completed.

2.2 Methods of abortion

Summary

The most appropriate methods of abortion differ by the duration of pregnancy. The methods summarized are indicative rather than prescriptive with regard to the time limits. For example, most trained providers can safely undertake vacuum aspiration up to 12 weeks of pregnancy, while others with sufficient experience and access to appropriately sized cannulae can use this procedure safely for terminating pregnancies of less than 15 weeks' duration (3).

The availability of safe and effective medical methods of inducing abortion has expanded due to the increased registration and use of mifepristone and misoprostol (global maps of registration of mifepristone and misoprostol are available at: www.gynuity.org). The knowledge of and correct use of these drugs, including that of misoprostol alone when mifepristone is not available, is important for programme planners, managers, health-care workers and pharmacists, as these drugs are introduced into health systems.

Methods up to 12–14 weeks since the last menstrual period

The recommended abortion methods are manual or electric vacuum aspiration, or medical methods using a combination of mifepristone followed by misoprostol.

Mifepristone followed by a prostaglandin analogue has been shown to be safe and effective up to 9 weeks (63 days) of pregnancy (*4, 19*). Limited evidence also suggests the safety and effectiveness of a regimen with repeated doses of misoprostol between 9 and 12 weeks of gestation (*3, 4, 27, 28*); however, misoprostol alone is less effective than its use in combination with mifepristone.

The use of medical methods of abortion requires the back-up of vacuum aspiration, either on-site or through referral to another health-care facility in case of failed or incomplete abortion.

Programme managers and policy-makers should make all possible efforts to replace D&C with vacuum aspiration and medical methods of abortion.

Methods after 12–14 weeks since the last menstrual period

The recommended surgical method is D&E, using vacuum aspiration and forceps. The recommended medical method for abortions after 12 weeks since the LMP is mifepristone followed by repeated doses of misoprostol.

Pre-procedure considerations

2.2.1 Cervical preparation

Cervical preparation (or priming) using osmotic dilators, such as laminaria, or pharmacological agents is commonly used before some first-trimester surgical abortions because it may make the abortion procedure quicker and easier to perform by reducing the need for mechanical cervical dilatation (*29, 30*). Cervical preparation before surgical abortion is especially beneficial for women with cervical anomalies or previous surgery, adolescents and those with advanced pregnancies, all of whom have a higher risk of cervical injury or uterine perforation that may cause haemorrhage (*31, 32*). It may also facilitate the abortion procedure for inexperienced providers. However, cervical preparation has disadvantages, including additional discomfort for the woman, and the extra cost and time required to administer it effectively. It is therefore recommended for all women with durations of pregnancy over 12–14 weeks (*29, 30, 33*), although its use may be considered for women at any gestational age, in particular those at high risk for cervical injury or uterine perforation.

Cervical preparation using osmotic dilators requires at least 4 hours to be effective. In first-trimester surgical abortion, research suggests that administration of 400 μg misoprostol either vaginally 3–4 hours or sublingually 2–3 hours prior to the procedure is effective in preparing the cervix (*29*). Another effective pharmacological regimen is 200 mg mifepristone taken orally 36 hours before a vacuum aspiration procedure (*29, 34*). For cervical priming prior to D&E, misoprostol is inferior to overnight dilatation with laminaria. Unlike laminaria, misoprostol used alone for cervical preparation has not been studied after 20 weeks' gestation. Misoprostol use in combination with overnight osmotic dilators does not have any additional benefit in cervical dilatation before 19 weeks of gestation (*30*).

2.2.2 Pain management

Most women report some degree of pain with abortion. The factors associated with pain during surgical abortion with local anaesthesia have been evaluated in several observational studies. The degree of the pain varies with the age of the woman, parity, history of dysmenorrhoea and the anxiety level or fearfulness of the woman (35–37). Prior vaginal delivery and greater experience of the provider have been found to be associated with less pain during abortion (35, 38). The relationship between pain and gestational age as well as the amount of cervical dilatation required for the abortion have shown conflicting results (35, 36, 38), although a shorter procedure time has been associated with less pain (35).

Providing adequate pain management does not require a large investment in drugs, equipment or training. Neglecting this important element needlessly increases women's anxiety and discomfort, thereby seriously compromising the quality of care and potentially increasing the difficulty of performing the procedure.

Counselling and sympathetic treatment may reduce women's fears and perceptions of pain, as has been reported for women treated for incomplete abortion (39). Non-pharmacological relaxation techniques can result in shorter procedure times and decreased need for pain medications (40, 41), and listening to music may decrease procedural pain (37). The person performing the procedure, and other staff present, should be friendly and reassuring. Where feasible, and if the woman wishes, it may also be helpful for a supportive person, such as the woman's husband or partner, a family member or friend, to remain with her during the procedure. However, non-pharmacological approaches should not be seen as a replacement for pharmacological pain alleviation.

2.2.2.1 Medication for pain

Medication for pain management should always be offered for both medical and surgical methods of abortion, and provided without delay to women who desire it. Three types of drugs, either singly or in combination, are used to manage pain during abortion: analgesics, which alleviate the sensation of pain; tranquillizers, which reduce anxiety; and anaesthetics, which decrease physical sensation during surgical abortion. In most cases of surgical abortion, analgesics, local anaesthesia and/or mild sedation supplemented by verbal reassurance, are sufficient. Most of these drugs are comparatively inexpensive.

Non-narcotic analgesics included on the *WHO Model list of essential medicines*, such as non-steroidal anti-inflammatory agents like ibuprofen, reduce pain, including uterine cramping, associated with both surgical and medical methods of abortion (42, 43). Paracetamol was found, in randomized controlled trials, to be ineffective to relieve post-procedural pain following surgical abortion (44–46) and was similarly ineffective at reducing pain during medical abortion (47); therefore, the use of paracetamol is not recommended to decrease pain during abortion.

For surgical abortion, preoperative administration of tranquillizers, such as diazepam, can reduce fear and induce relaxation, making the procedure easier for both the woman and the provider. Such drugs can cause amnesia, which some women may want, but they may also induce drowsiness and delay ambulation (37). Supplemental use of narcotic analgesics may also be appropriate, though the possibility of complications such as respiratory depression means that resuscitation capability and narcotic-reversal agents must be available.

2.2.2.2 Anaesthesia

Where mechanical cervical dilatation is required for surgical abortion, a paracervical block using a local anaesthetic, such as rapidly acting lidocaine, injected beneath the cervical mucosa around the cervix, is commonly used. Advantages of using local rather than general anaesthesia include a reduction in procedural risks and complications, a faster recovery time, and a greater sense of control for the woman, who remains conscious and able to communicate with the provider. Injection of local anaesthetic must be done skilfully, to avoid intravenous introduction of the drug. The use of local anaesthesia with vacuum aspiration is safe; however, the degree to which it decreases pain has not been well studied, despite its common use (37).

General anaesthesia is not routinely recommended for abortion procedures, and increases the clinical risks (1, 48–50). It has been associated with higher rates of haemorrhage than local anaesthesia (1, 2). Use of general anaesthesia increases costs for both the health-care facility and the woman, particularly as some hospital policies unnecessarily require women who receive it to stay overnight. Nevertheless, as it is the most effective method of pain control, some women prefer general anaesthesia, and its use may also be preferable from the provider's perspective during difficult procedures. Any facility that offers general anaesthesia must have the specialized equipment and staff to administer it and to handle any complications.

2.2.3 Induction of pre-procedure fetal demise

When using medical methods of abortion after 20 weeks' gestation, inducing pre-procedure fetal demise should be considered. Modern medical methods, such as combination regimens of mifepristone and misoprostol or misoprostol alone, are not directly feticidal; the incidence of transient fetal survival after expulsion is related to increasing gestational age and decreasing interval to abortion (51, 52). Commonly used pre-procedure regimens to effect fetal demise include (53):

- Injection of potassium chloride (KCl) through the fetal umbilical cord or into the fetal cardiac chambers, which is highly effective but requires

expertise for precise, safe injection and time to observe cardiac cessation on ultrasound.

- Intra-amniotic or intrafetal injection of digoxin. Digoxin has a higher failure rate than KCl to cause intrauterine fetal demise; however, it is technically easier to use, does not require ultrasound if administered intra-amniotically, and has demonstrated safety (maternal serum levels remain at or below therapeutic digoxin levels) (51). Digoxin requires time for fetal absorption; therefore, it is commonly administered the day before induction of abortion with misoprostol (33, 54).

2.2.4 Surgical methods of abortion

2.2.4.1 Vacuum aspiration

The recommended surgical technique for abortion up to gestational age less than 15 weeks is vacuum aspiration (57). The high efficacy of vacuum aspiration has been well established in several randomized controlled trials. Complete abortion rates between 95% and 100% are reported (55, 56). Electric and manual vacuum technologies appear to be equally effective; however, the use of manual vacuum aspiration is associated with less pain in pregnancies under 9 weeks' gestation and with more procedural difficulty over 9 weeks' gestation (57). Vacuum aspiration under 14 weeks' gestation is more effective and associated with fewer minor complications than medical abortion (56, 58).

Vacuum aspiration involves evacuation of the contents of the uterus through a plastic or metal cannula, attached to a vacuum source. Electric vacuum aspiration (EVA) employs an electric vacuum pump. With manual vacuum aspiration (MVA), the vacuum is created using a hand-held, hand-activated, plastic 60 ml aspirator (also called a syringe). Available aspirators accommodate different sizes of plastic cannulae, ranging from 4 mm to 16 mm in diameter. For each procedure, the appropriately sized cannula should be chosen based on the gestational age and the amount of cervical dilatation present; generally, the diameter of the cannula corresponds to the gestational age in weeks. Some cannulae and most aspirators are reusable after being cleaned and high-level disinfected or sterilized. Foot-operated mechanical pumps are also available.

Depending on the duration of pregnancy, abortion with vacuum aspiration takes from 3 to 10 minutes to complete and can be performed on an outpatient basis, using analgesics and/or local anaesthesia. The completion of abortion is verified by examination of the aspirated tissue. In very early pregnancy, the cannula may be inserted without prior dilatation of the cervix. Usually, however, dilatation using mechanical or osmotic dilators, or pharmacological agents such as misoprostol or mifepristone, is required before insertion of the cannula (see Section 2.2.1). Generally, vacuum-aspiration procedures can be safely completed without intrauterine use of curettes or other instruments. No data suggest that use of curettage after vacuum aspiration decreases the risk of retained products (59).

Most women who have a first-trimester abortion with local anaesthesia feel well enough to leave the health-care facility after observation for about 30 minutes in a recovery room. Longer recovery periods are generally needed for abortions performed later in pregnancy and when sedation or general anaesthesia has been used.

Vacuum aspiration is a very safe procedure. A study of 170 000 first-trimester abortions conducted in New York City by vacuum aspiration reported that less than 0.1% of the women experienced serious complications requiring hospitalization (60). Though rare, complications with vacuum aspiration can include pelvic infection, excessive bleeding, cervical injury, incomplete evacuation, uterine perforation, anaesthetic complications and ongoing pregnancy (1, 2). Abdominal cramping and menstrual-like bleeding occur with any abortion procedure.

2.2.4.2 Dilatation and curettage

D&C involves dilating the cervix with mechanical dilators or pharmacological agents and using sharp metal curettes to scrape the walls of the uterus.

D&C is less safe than vacuum aspiration (61) and considerably more painful for women (62). Therefore, vacuum aspiration should replace D&C. The rates of major complications of D&C are two to three times higher than those of vacuum aspiration (3). Randomized controlled trials comparing D&C with vacuum aspiration found that, for up to 10 weeks since the LMP, vacuum aspiration is quicker and associated with less blood loss than D&C (63, 64).

Where it is still practised, all possible efforts should be made to replace D&C with vacuum aspiration, to improve the safety and quality of care for women. Where no abortion services are currently offered, vacuum aspiration should be introduced rather than D&C. At sites where vacuum aspiration has yet to be introduced, managers must ensure that proper pain-management protocols are followed, and that D&C procedures are performed by well-trained staff under adequate supervision.

2.2.4.3 Dilatation and evacuation

D&E is used after 12–14 weeks of pregnancy. It is the safest and most effective surgical technique for later abortion, where skilled, experienced providers are available (3). D&E requires preparation of the cervix using osmotic dilators or pharmacological agents (see Section 2.1) and evacuating the uterus using EVA with 12–16 mm diameter cannulae and long forceps. Depending on the duration of pregnancy, preparation to achieve adequate cervical dilatation can require from 2 hours to 2 days. Many providers find the use of ultrasound helpful during D&E procedures, but its use is not essential (65).

A randomized controlled trial comparing D&E with intra-amniotic instillation of prostaglandin $PGF_{2\alpha}$ found D&E to be faster, safer and more acceptable, at least up to 18 weeks of pregnancy (66). D&E has been compared to the use of mifepristone with repeated doses of misoprostol in one small trial, where it was found to be associated with less pain and fewer adverse events (67). Like any medical procedure, providers need the requisite training, equipment and skills to safely perform D&E (68).

A D&E procedure can usually be performed on an outpatient basis with a paracervical block and non-steroidal anti-inflammatory analgesics or conscious sedation. General anaesthesia is not required and can increase risk (see Section 2.2.2.2). A D&E procedure usually takes no more than 30 minutes to perform. Clinic staff and women undergoing the procedure should expect more postoperative vaginal bleeding than after a first-trimester abortion. Staff should also be trained to provide counselling and information specific to second-trimester abortion.

2.2.4.4 Other surgical methods of abortion for use in later pregnancy

Major surgical operations should not be used as primary methods of abortion. Hysterotomy has no role in contemporary abortion practice, since its morbidity, mortality and cost are markedly higher than those of D&E or medical methods of abortion. Similarly, hysterectomy should not be used except for women with conditions that would warrant the operation independently (19).

2.2.4.5 Tissue examination following surgical abortion

After surgical methods of abortion, immediate examination of the products of conception is important to exclude the possibility of ectopic pregnancy and assess whether the abortion is likely to be complete. With vacuum aspiration, beginning around 6 weeks of pregnancy, trained providers can visually identify the products of conception, specifically chorionic villi and the gestational sac (59). If the aspirate does not contain products of conception, ectopic pregnancy should be suspected and the woman should undergo further evaluation (see Section 2.1.6). In addition, providers should be alert to tissue appearances suggestive of molar pregnancy, particularly in countries where molar pregnancy is common. If the contents of the aspirate contain less tissue than expected, the possibility of incomplete abortion and treatment with re-aspiration should be considered. Routine examination of the products of conception by a pathology laboratory is not necessary when trained providers perform routine tissue examination.

2.2.5 Medical methods of abortion (see Box 2.1)

Medical methods of abortion have been proved to be safe and effective (4, 19, 24, 69–71). The most effective regimens rely on the antiprogestogen, mifepristone, which binds to progesterone receptors, inhibiting the action of progesterone and hence interfering with the continuation of pregnancy. Treatment regimens entail an initial dose of mifepristone followed by administration of a synthetic prostaglandin analogue, generally misoprostol, which enhances uterine contractions and aids in expelling the products of conception (72). Gemeprost is a prostaglandin analogue similar to misoprostol, but it is more expensive, requires refrigeration, and may only be administered vaginally (12). Thus, although

BOX 2.1

Dosages and routes of administration for mifepristone followed by misoprostol

For pregnancies of gestational age up to 9 weeks (63 days)

- 200 mg **mifepristone** administered orally.
- Administration of **misoprostol** is recommended 1 to 2 days (24–48 hours) following ingestion of mifepristone.
- For vaginal, buccal or sublingual routes, the recommended dose of misoprostol is 800 µg.
- For oral administration, the recommended dose of misoprostol is 400 µg.
- With gestations up to **7 weeks** (49 days) misoprostol may be administered by vaginal, buccal, sublingual or oral routes. After 7 weeks of gestation, oral administration of misoprostol should *not* be used.
- With gestations up to **9 weeks** (63 days) misoprostol can be administered by vaginal, buccal or sublingual routes.

For pregnancies of gestational age 9–12 weeks (63–84 days)

- 200 mg **mifepristone** administered orally, followed after 36 to 48 hours by:
- 800 µg vaginal **misoprostol**, administered in a health-care facility. A maximum of four further doses of misoprostol 400 µg may be administered at 3-hourly intervals, vaginally or sublingually.

For pregnancies of gestational age over 12 weeks (>84 days)

- 200 mg mifepristone administered orally, followed after 36 to 48 hours by:
- 400 µg oral or 800 µg vaginal misoprostol followed by 400 µg vaginal or sublingual misoprostol every 3 hours up to a maximum of five doses, administered in a health-care facility. For pregnancies of gestational age greater than 24 weeks, the dose of misoprostol should be reduced due to the greater sensitivity of the uterus to prostaglandins, but the lack of clinical studies precludes specific dosing recommendations.

gemeprost demonstrates similar efficacy as misoprostol, misoprostol is the prostaglandin analogue of choice for abortion-related care (*73*). A number of other prostaglandins that were used in the past, such as sulprostone and prostaglandin $F_{2\alpha}$, are no longer used because of their adverse side-effects or relative lack of efficacy (*74*).

The effects of medical methods of abortion are similar to those associated with spontaneous abortion and include uterine cramping and prolonged menstrual-like bleeding. Bleeding occurs for 9 days on average but can last up to 45 days in rare cases (*75*).

Side-effects include nausea, vomiting and diarrhoea. Contraindications to the use of mifepristone and a prostaglandin analogue include chronic or acute adrenal or hepatic failure, inherited porphyria, and allergy to any of the drugs used. Mifepristone is not an effective treatment for ectopic pregnancy; suspicion of ectopic pregnancy demands further investigation and, if confirmed, immediate treatment (*11*). Caution and clinical judgement are required for women using corticosteroids long term, and for those who have bleeding disorders, severe anaemia, pre-existing heart disease or cardiovascular risk factors (*12*).

Medical methods of abortion have proved acceptable in many settings, including low-resource settings (76–78). The medications are increasingly available globally, and the combination of mifepristone and misoprostol for medical abortion is now included on the *WHO model list of essential medicines* (73, 79). As these medications become increasingly available, programme managers should be aware of what is required to introduce medical methods of abortion into existing health services (see Chapter 3).

2.2.5.1 Mifepristone and prostaglandin analogue

For pregnancies of gestational age up to 9 weeks (63 days)

Mifepristone with misoprostol has been proven highly effective, safe and acceptable for abortions occurring up to 9 weeks since the LMP. Efficacy rates up to 98% are reported (70, 80). Approximately 2–5% of women treated with the combination of mifepristone and misoprostol will require surgical intervention to resolve an incomplete abortion, terminate a continuing pregnancy, or control bleeding (81).

The original protocols for the use of mifepristone recommended an oral dose of 600 mg mifepristone followed by 1 mg of vaginal gemeprost after 36–48 hours. However, several studies have established that 200 mg of mifepristone is the dosage of choice, since it is as effective as 600 mg, and reduces costs when followed by a suitable prostaglandin analogue (4, 81–83). Some studies have indicated that mifepristone can be given as five or six divided doses of 25 mg over 3 days, for a total dose of 125–150 mg (84), a regimen widely used in the People's Republic of China. However, for service delivery and patient convenience, the single dose of mifepristone is recommended. A 50 mg dose of mifepristone is less effective than 200 mg, when given in combination with gemeprost (85). One trial reported that mifepristone, 100 mg, when combined with

800 µg of misoprostol given vaginally, was as effective as 200 mg; however, efficacy in both arms of this study was lower than expected (86).

Misoprostol is an effective prostaglandin analogue that is considerably less expensive than gemeprost, and does not require refrigeration. It is therefore the prostaglandin analogue of choice. An oral dose of 200 mg mifepristone followed by 800 µg misoprostol administered vaginally, sublingually or buccally is an effective medical abortion regimen (4). When compared to vaginal administration, sublingual misoprostol appears to be associated with higher rates of gastrointestinal side-effects, and buccal administration appears to be associated with higher rates of diarrhoea (4). Vaginal misoprostol is more effective and better tolerated than misoprostol given orally (87). Misoprostol given orally at a dose of 400 µg should be restricted to pregnancies up to 7 weeks' (49 days') gestation, given its higher failure rate when given orally as pregnancy progresses (12, 81).

Some protocols require that women take both mifepristone and a prostaglandin analogue under clinical supervision, involving a second visit to the health-care facility one or two days after receiving mifepristone, to take the prostaglandin analogue. Home use of misoprostol is a safe option for women (80, 88). Increasingly, after receiving the mifepristone in the clinic, women receive misoprostol for self-administration at home within 24–48 hours following the mifepristone. Nevertheless, some women may prefer clinic use (89). Women using misoprostol at home may leave the facility shortly after taking the mifepristone. They must be told what to expect with regard to vaginal bleeding and expulsion of products of conception following use of misoprostol, and how to recognize complications and whom to contact if they should occur. Explaining that the misoprostol dose should be taken as planned regardless of whether

Clinical care for women undergoing abortion

bleeding occurs following mifepristone is important for the few women who experience such bleeding.

Following administration of the misoprostol, up to 90% of women will expel the products of conception over the following 4–6 hours. Most women are likely to require medication for cramping pain during this period of time (see Section 2.2.2.1).

In the case of a failed abortion where pregnancy is ongoing, re-administration of misoprostol or surgical abortion should be offered to the woman (12). Women with incomplete abortions can generally be observed unless vaginal bleeding is heavy, or they may be offered re-administration of misoprostol or surgical completion of their abortion. Facilities offering medical methods of abortion must be able to ensure provision of vacuum aspiration, if needed. Such provision can be available on-site or through an arrangement with another facility that performs vacuum aspiration. In all cases, health-care providers must ensure that the woman can reach such services in case of an emergency.

Women are more likely to be satisfied with the procedure if they have realistic expectations about the abortion process (90). Hence, they need complete information about what is to be expected with, and the possible side-effects of, medical methods of abortion. Health-care workers should ensure that women understand the importance of complying with the protocol, especially for drugs that are self-administered, and that they know how to recognize, and what to do in case of, complications.

For pregnancies of gestational age from 9 to 12 weeks (63–84 days)
Limited data suggest that during this period the most effective medical regimen is mifepristone 200 mg orally followed 36–48 hours later by misoprostol 800 µg vaginally, administered in a health-care

facility. A maximum of four further doses of misoprostol 400 µg may be administered at three-hourly intervals, vaginally or sublingually (27, 28). Regimens during this period of pregnancy and the setting in which they can be administered are the subject of ongoing research.

For pregnancies of gestational age over 12 weeks (>84 days)
A regimen of oral mifepristone, 200 mg, followed by repeated doses of misoprostol is safe and highly effective when administered in a health-care facility (3, 91). An oral dose of 200 mg mifepristone followed 36–48 hours later by an initial dose of misoprostol, either 400 µg orally or 800 µg vaginally, with further doses of 400 µg of vaginal or sublingual misoprostol every 3 hours, up to four further doses is highly effective (91). For pregnancies beyond 24 weeks' gestation, the dose of misoprostol should be reduced, due to the greater sensitivity of the uterus to prostaglandins, but the lack of clinical studies precludes specific dosing recommendations.

A vaginally administered dose of 1 mg gemeprost used after 200 mg mifepristone, and repeated if necessary every 6 hours up to four doses can also be used effectively (92). The treatment with gemeprost may continue with 1 mg gemeprost every 3 hours for four additional doses if necessary (93, 94).

2.2.5.2 Misoprostol alone

For pregnancies of gestational age up to 12 weeks (84 days)
Misoprostol alone has also been studied for medical abortion in terms of effectiveness and safety. The effectiveness of misoprostol alone is lower, the time to complete abortion is prolonged, and the abortion process is more painful and associated with higher rates of gastrointestinal side-effects than when misoprostol is combined with mifepristone

(*4*, *95*). Because of misoprostol's wide availability and low cost, and since in some settings its broader use has been reported to contribute to a decrease in complications from unsafe abortion (*96*), the use of misoprostol alone appears to be common where mifepristone is unavailable.

The recommended misoprostol regimens are 800 µg administered vaginally or sublingually, and repeated at intervals no less than 3 hours but no more than 12 hours for up to three doses. This regimen is 75–90% effective in completing abortion. Sublingual administration is less effective than vaginal administration unless it is given every 3 hours, but this regimen has high rates of gastrointestinal side-effects (*4*, *96*, *97*). Oral administration is not recommended due to its low efficacy.

For pregnancies of gestational age over 12 weeks (84 days)

Misoprostol is effective in inducing abortion after 12 weeks of pregnancy, although the time to complete abortion is not as short as when it is used in combination with mifepristone. The recommended regimen is 400 µg of vaginal or sublingual misoprostol every 3 hours for up to five doses (*91*, *98*). Particularly for nulliparous women, vaginal administration of misoprostol is more effective than sublingual dosing. For pregnancies beyond 24 weeks' gestation, the dose of misoprostol should be reduced due to the greater sensitivity of the uterus to prostaglandins; however, the lack of clinical studies precludes dosing recommendations.

Vaginal administration of gemeprost alone is registered for termination of second-trimester pregnancy in several countries. The recommended dose is 1 mg, which is given every 3 hours up to five times during the first day and repeated the next day if necessary. With this treatment, 80% and 95% of women will abort within 24 and 48 hours, respectively (*99*).

2.2.5.3 Other medical abortion agents

Methotrexate, which is a cytotoxic drug used to treat certain types of cancer, rheumatoid arthritis, psoriasis and some other conditions, has been used in combination with misoprostol as a medical method for early abortion (pregnancies of gestational age up to 7 weeks) in some countries where mifepristone has not been available. When combined with misoprostol, it is effective: a number of studies report an overall success rate of greater than 90% with 50 mg of methotrexate orally or intramuscularly, followed by 800 µg vaginal misoprostol 3–7 days later (*4*). However, a WHO toxicology panel recommended against the use of methotrexate for inducing abortion, based on concerns of teratogenicity if the pregnancy was not successfully aborted (*100*). Although the actual risks are as yet unknown, limb defects and skull and facial abnormalities in pregnancies that continued after failed attempts to induce abortion with methotrexate have been reported (*101–103*). It is therefore recommended that services wishing to introduce medical methods of abortion use combination regimens of mifepristone and misoprostol.

Other agents are used to stimulate uterine contractions and induce abortion after 12 weeks, but available data regarding their safety are limited. These agents include hypertonic saline, or hyperosmolar urea, injected intra-amniotically; ethacridine lactate administered intra- or extra-amniotically; prostaglandin analogues administered parenterally or intra- or extra-amniotically; and oxytocin injected intravenously or intramuscularly (*91*, *104*). These methods and routes of administration, however, are invasive and likely to be less safe, and the time to complete abortion is longer when compared to the use of methods such as combined mifepristone and misoprostol.

Clinical care for women undergoing abortion

2.2.6 Managing abortion complications

When abortion is performed by appropriately trained personnel under modern medical conditions, complications are impressively rare and the risk of death is negligible (in contrast to unsafe abortion, see Chapter 1). Nevertheless, every service-delivery site at each level of the health system should be equipped and have personnel trained to recognize abortion complications and to provide, or refer women for, prompt care, 24 hours a day (*104*). The facilities and skills required to manage most abortion complications are similar to those needed to care for women who have had a spontaneous abortion (miscarriage).

2.2.6.1 Ongoing pregnancy

Failed abortion with ongoing pregnancy can occur in women who have undergone either surgical or medical methods of abortion, although it is more common after medical procedures. Women with continuing symptoms of pregnancy or clinical signs of failed abortion should be offered a uterine evacuation procedure as expeditiously as possible (*19*).

2.2.6.2 Incomplete abortion

Incomplete abortion is uncommon following vacuum aspiration when the abortion is performed by a skilled provider. It is more common with medical methods of abortion (*56*). Common symptoms include vaginal bleeding and abdominal pain, and signs of infection may be present. Incomplete abortion should also be suspected if, upon visual examination, the tissue aspirated during surgical abortion is not compatible with the estimated duration of pregnancy. Staff at every health-care facility should be trained and equipped to treat incomplete abortion by emptying the uterus, paying attention to the possibility of haemorrhage, which might cause anaemia, or infection, which would necessitate antibiotic treatment.

Incomplete abortion may be treated using either vacuum aspiration or misoprostol. Vacuum aspiration is recommended over D&C for uterine evacuation, as it is associated with less blood loss, less pain and shorter procedure times (*105*). Incomplete abortion may also be treated using misoprostol: no differences were demonstrated in rates of complete abortion or of adverse events between uterine aspiration or misoprostol for women with incomplete spontaneous abortion (miscarriage) with uterine size up to 13 weeks' gestation, although there were more unplanned surgical interventions with misoprostol use (*106*). The recommended misoprostol dose and route of administration for this indication is either 600 µg oral or 400 µg sublingual (*106, 107*). The presence of bleeding may decrease misoprostol absorption when the drug is administered vaginally (*108*); thus, a non-vaginal route is generally preferable, although vaginal administration of 400–800 µg has been used effectively (*106*). Incomplete spontaneous abortions may also be managed expectantly, for women who are clinically stable and wish to avoid medical or surgical treatment, but the process takes more time (*106*). The decision about management of incomplete abortion should be based upon the clinical condition of the woman and her preference for treatment.

2.2.6.3 Haemorrhage

Haemorrhage can result from retained products of conception, trauma or damage to the cervix, coagulopathy or, rarely, uterine perforation. Depending on the cause of the haemorrhage, appropriate treatment may include re-evacuation of the uterus and administration of uterotonic drugs to stop the bleeding, intravenous fluid replacement, and, in severe cases, blood transfusion, replacement of clotting factors, laparoscopy or exploratory laparotomy. Because of the low incidence of haemorrhage using vacuum aspiration, oxytocic drugs are not routinely needed, although they may be indicated with D&E. Prolonged menstrual-like bleeding is an expected effect of medical methods of abortion. On average, vaginal bleeding gradually diminishes over about 2 weeks after medical abortion but, in individual cases, bleeding and spotting may persist for up to 45 days; such bleeding is rarely heavy enough to constitute an emergency. Surgical evacuation may be performed on the woman's request, or in cases where the bleeding is heavy or prolonged, causes anaemia, or there is evidence of infection. However, every service-delivery site must be able to stabilize and treat or refer women with haemorrhage immediately (19).

2.2.6.4 Infection

Infection rarely occurs following properly performed abortions. The genital tract, however, is more susceptible to ascending infection when the cervix is dilated after abortion or childbirth. Common signs and symptoms of infection include fever or chills, foul-smelling vaginal or cervical discharge, abdominal or pelvic pain, prolonged vaginal bleeding or spotting, uterine tenderness, and/or an elevated white blood cell count. When infection is diagnosed, health-care staff should administer antibiotics and, if retained products of conception are a likely cause of the infection, re-evacuate the uterus. Women with severe infections may require hospitalization. As discussed in Section 2.1.5, prophylactic provision of antibiotics for women undergoing surgical abortion has been found to reduce the risk of post-abortion infection (9) and they should be provided where possible.

There are few data on the incidence of clinically significant pelvic infection after medical abortion, but it occurs rarely and possibly less frequently than after vacuum aspiration. Many of the symptoms of pelvic infection, such as pain, are rather nonspecific and hence precise diagnosis is difficult. Women with pelvic pain, abdominal or adnexal tenderness, vaginal discharge, and fever should be treated with broad-spectrum antibiotics.

Rare cases of anaerobic infection without fever have been reported from Canada and the USA, following medical abortion (10, 12, 109). No such cases have been reported elsewhere. In these cases, women had little or no fever; variable nausea, vomiting, weakness and some abdominal pain; rapid deterioration within hours or days; tachycardia and refractory hypotension; multiple effusions; elevated haematocrit; and elevated leukocyte count and neutrophilia. All women had Clostridium-related toxic shock. Reported cases have also occurred outside of abortion care, such as during the postpartum period following a normal delivery (110). There is no evidence that prophylactic antibiotic treatment during medical abortion would eliminate these rare fatal cases of serious infection; therefore, prophylactic provision of antibiotics for women undergoing medical abortion is not recommended.

2.2.6.5 Uterine perforation

Uterine perforation usually goes undetected and resolves without the need for intervention. A study of more than 700 women undergoing concurrent first-trimester abortion and laparoscopic sterilization found that 12 out of the 14 uterine perforations were so small that they would not have been recognized had laparoscopy not been performed (111). When uterine perforation is suspected, observation and antibiotic treatment may be all that is necessary. When available and necessary, laparoscopy is the investigative method of choice. If the laparoscopy examination and/or the status of the patient give rise to any suspicion of damage to the bowel, blood vessels or other structures, a laparotomy to repair the damaged structures may be needed.

2.2.6.6 Anaesthesia-related complications

Local anaesthesia is safer than general anaesthesia, both for vacuum aspiration in the first trimester and for D&E in the second trimester (1, 49, 50). Where general anaesthesia is used, staff must be skilled in management of seizures and cardiorespiratory resuscitation. Narcotic-reversal agents should always be readily available in settings where narcotics are used.

2.2.6.7 Uterine rupture

Uterine rupture is a rare complication. It is associated with later gestational ages and uterine scar, but has also been reported in women without these risk factors. In a meta-analysis, the risk of uterine rupture in women with a prior caesarean delivery having a misoprostol-induced abortion in the second trimester was found to be 0.28% (112).

2.2.6.8 Long-term sequelae

The vast majority of women who have a properly performed induced abortion will not suffer any long-term effects on their general or reproductive health (113–115). In modern times, the risk of death from a safe, induced abortion is lower than from an injection of penicillin (116) or carrying a pregnancy to term (1).

Research shows no association between safely induced first-trimester abortion and adverse outcomes in subsequent pregnancies (117). Although second-trimester abortions have not been studied as extensively, there is no evidence of an increased risk of adverse outcomes in subsequent pregnancies (114, 118). Sound epidemiological data show no increased risk of breast cancer for women following spontaneous or induced abortion (119, 120). Negative psychological sequelae occur in a very small number of women and appear to be the continuation of pre-existing conditions, rather than being a result of the experience of induced abortion (121, 122).

2.2.6.9 Other complications

Following unsafe abortion, various other complications may occur that result from the manner or method of provoking the abortion. Examples are poisoning, abdominal trauma, or the presence of foreign bodies in the genital tract, among others. Women with these complications should be stabilized and treated or referred for appropriate treatment, in addition to managing any abortion-related complications (see Sections 2.2.6.1–2.2.6.6) and receiving appropriate post-procedure care (see Section 2.3).

2.2.7 Other issues related to abortion procedures

2.2.7.1 Infection prevention and control

Since abortion procedures and care involve contact with blood and other body fluids, all clinical and support staff in all facilities that provide these services should understand and apply standard precautions for infection prevention and control, for both their own protection and that of their patients.

Standard precautions are simple infection-control practices to be used in the care of all patients, at all times, to reduce the risk of transmission of blood-borne infections. They include: hand-washing with soap and water before and after all procedures; use of protective barriers such as gloves, gowns, aprons, masks, and goggles to avoid direct contact with blood and other body fluids; safe disposal of waste contaminated with blood or other body fluids; proper handling of soiled linen; careful handling and disposal of "sharps"; and proper disinfection of instruments and other contaminated equipment (123).

Hand-washing and use of protective barriers

All staff should wash their hands thoroughly before and after coming into contact with the woman, as well as immediately following any contact with blood, body fluids or mucous membranes (*124*). High-level disinfected or sterile gloves should be worn and replaced between contacts with different patients and between vaginal (or rectal) examinations of the same woman. After completing the care of one woman and removing gloves, the health-care provider should always wash their hands, as gloves may have undetected holes in them (*124*). The use of auxiliary supplies, such as sterile booties, does not make a significant difference in infection rates, although it increases costs.

Cleaning

Detergents and hot water are adequate for the routine cleaning of floors, beds, toilets, walls, and rubber draw sheets. Following spillage of body fluids, heavy-duty rubber gloves should be worn and as much body fluid as possible removed with an absorbent material. This can then be discarded in a leak-proof container and later incinerated or buried in a deep pit. The area of spillage should be cleaned with a chlorine-based disinfectant and then thoroughly washed with hot soap and water.

All soiled linen should be handled as little as possible, bagged at the point of collection and not sorted or rinsed in patient-care areas. If possible, linen with large amounts of body fluid should be transported in leak-proof bags. If leak-proof bags are not available, the linen should be folded with the soiled parts inside, and handled carefully, wearing gloves.

Safe disposal of waste contaminated with body fluids

Solid waste that is contaminated with blood, body fluids, laboratory specimens or body tissue should be treated as clinical waste, and disposed of properly and in accordance with local regulations (*123*). Liquid waste, such as blood or other body fluids, should be poured down a drain connected to an adequately treated sewer or pit latrine.

Safe handling and disposal of "sharps"

The greatest hazard of HIV transmission in health-care settings is through skin puncture with contaminated needles or "sharps". This also applies to transmission of hepatitis B and C. Most "sharps" injuries involving such transmission are through deep injuries with hollow-bore needles. Such injuries frequently occur when needles are recapped, cleaned, disposed of, or inappropriately discarded. Although recapping needles is to be avoided whenever possible (*124*), sometimes recapping is necessary. When this is the case, a single-handed scooping method should be used. Puncture-resistant disposal containers must be available and readily accessible for the disposal of "sharps". These can be burned in a closed incinerator or buried in a deep pit. Added precautions to prevent "sharps" injuries include wearing gloves, having an adequate light source when treating women, placing "sharps" containers directly at the point of use, never discarding "sharps" in general waste, and keeping "sharps" out of the reach of children. Whenever possible, needle holders should be used when suturing.

Safe cleaning of equipment after use

Immediately after use, all reusable surgical instruments used in abortion should be sent for cleaning and sterilization. Medical equipment and supplies intended for single use should not be reused (*124*). Where central services for instrument processing are not available, or in resource-poor settings, the following procedures are recommended.

The most important step to ensure proper final decontamination of instruments is physical cleaning

(123). Instruments should be kept wet until cleaning. Letting the devices dry may make it difficult to completely remove all contaminants. A disinfectant such as a 0.5% chlorine solution can be used. Aspirators must be disassembled before cleaning and further processing. Detachable adaptors must be removed from cannulae.

> Caution: aspirators, cannulae and adaptors are not safe to handle with bare hands until cleaned.

After soaking, wash all surfaces thoroughly in running water and detergent. Detergent is preferable to soap, which can leave a residue. All instruments should then be sterilized (preferred) or disinfected with a high-level disinfectant (where sterilization is not possible or feasible). Sterilization kills all microorganisms, including bacterial endospores such as those that cause tetanus and gas-gangrene. High-level disinfection (HLD) destroys all microorganisms including hepatitis and HIV but does not reliably kill bacterial endospores.

Sterilization is best achieved with pressurized steam (autoclave) or multi-hour (>5 hours) soaks in fresh glutaraldehyde solution (125). HLD can be achieved by shorter soaks in glutaraldehyde or bleach (sodium hypochlorite) solutions (125). The use of phenol or antiseptics will not achieve HLD. Instruments that were cold-processed (soaked in solutions) must be thoroughly rinsed after processing. Instruments that were subjected to HLD may be rinsed in boiled water; instruments that were sterilized should be rinsed in sterile water (see Table 2.1 for instrument-processing details).

Table 2.1 Instrument processing

Method	Agent	Time	Notes
Sterilization	Pressurized steam (autoclave)	20 minutes at 121°C and 103.5–140 kPa pressure	Assumes the areas of equipment targeted for decontamination are accessible to steam. Time should be increased to 30 minutes for wrapped items.
	2% glutaraldehyde	5 hours contact at 20–25°C with a 2% activated alkaline formulation (pH = 7.5–9)	Some sources/manufacturers suggest 10 hours for sterilization.
High-level disinfection (HLD)	Chlorine (sodium hypochlorite)	5 minutes contact at 20–25°C with buffered hypochlorite (pH = 7–8) at a concentration of 5000 ppm available chlorine (approximately 10% dilution of household bleach – can be corrosive to metals)	Some sources recommend 20 minutes in a 5% dilution if made with tap water, or 1% dilution if made with boiled water.
	2% glutaraldehyde	30 minutes contact at 20–25°C with a 2% activated alkaline formulation (pH = 7.5–9)	Some sources/manufacturers suggest 20 minutes for HLD.
	Boiling	20 minutes at a "rolling boil"	The pot should be covered; items that float do not need to be fully immersed.

Note: the effectiveness of all sterilization and HLD techniques depends on prior cleaning to remove organic matter or material that is dried and adherent to the equipment (123, 125, 126).

Some manufacturers produce aspirators and cannulae made of high-grade plastics that are engineered to be sterilized in an autoclave, while other plastic instruments will crack and melt when exposed to high heat for sterilization. Health-care workers should always refer to the instructions for use of all items being disinfected, to ensure they are using the appropriate form of disinfection. Additionally, the manufacturers' instructions for all products used in the disinfection process should be followed.

2.3 Post-abortion care and follow-up

Following an induced or spontaneous abortion, women should receive appropriate post-abortion care. For those women whose abortions were performed unsafely, post-abortion care is used as a strategy to attenuate the morbidity and mortality associated with complications, including uterine aspiration for incomplete abortion (see Section 2.2.6.2); offer of contraception to prevent future unintended pregnancies; and linking women with other needed services in the community. Following safe, induced abortion, post-abortion care may not require a follow-up visit if the woman has adequate information about when to seek care for complications and has received any needed supplies or information to meet her contraceptive needs.

All women should receive contraceptive information and be offered counselling for and methods of post-abortion contraception, including emergency contraception, before leaving the health-care facility. All methods of contraception, including IUDs and hormonal contraceptives, can be initiated immediately following surgical or medical abortion, as long as attention is paid to each woman's health profile and the limitations associated with certain methods (see Annex 6). There are a few methods that should

not be started immediately following an abortion: the contraceptive diaphragm and cervical cap should not be used until about 6 weeks after a second-trimester abortion, and fertility-awareness-based methods should only be started after the resumption of regular menses (127). IUDs placed immediately post-abortion offer better protection against unintended pregnancy than postponing insertion (128–130). Although it is safe, there is a higher risk of expulsion of IUDs if inserted at the time of a second-trimester abortion (131). For medical abortion, hormonal contraceptives can be started by the woman after taking the first pill of a medical abortion regimen, but confirmation that the abortion is complete should precede insertion of an IUD or sterilization. Additionally, special attention should be given when women request sterilization, to ensure their choice is not unduly influenced by the nature of the moment.

Abortion-service-delivery sites should be able to provide a woman's contraceptive method of choice in the facility. If the contraceptive method chosen by the woman cannot be provided on-site (e.g. sterilization is rarely offered at primary-care level), the woman should be given information about where and how she can obtain it, and be offered an interim method. For those methods not available on-site, the abortion facility should develop a direct referral system to ensure women are able to obtain their chosen contraceptive method. All women should be informed about emergency contraception, and consideration should be given to providing it to them to be kept at home for future use, particularly for women who choose condoms as their primary method of contraception and those who choose not to start using a routine contraceptive method immediately.

Providers should discuss prevention of STIs, including HIV, and the importance of condom use with women who choose methods other than condoms for contraception (*127*). Information about infection prevention should be particularly emphasized for individuals who may be at increased risk, and in areas of known high prevalence of HIV and other STIs. HIV counselling and testing should be available in the facility, or by referral to other facilities. Dual protection, or the use of one method such as condoms, or a combination of methods, to protect against both pregnancy and STIs should be promoted.

Women undergoing abortion should receive clear, simple, oral and written instructions about how to care for themselves after leaving the health-care facility, and how to recognize complications that require medical attention. These instructions should include: abstaining from sexual intercourse and from placing anything in the vagina until bleeding stops; the availability of contraception, including emergency contraception, to avoid a pregnancy (fertility may return as soon as 2 weeks following abortion); and the need to return to the health-care facility in case of increasing pelvic pain, heavy bleeding or fever (*19*). During the time it takes for a medical abortion to be completed, women should be able to contact, at any time, a physician or other health-care worker who can answer questions and provide support.

2.3.1 Surgical methods of abortion

During the observation period following surgical abortion, staff should offer women comfort and support and monitor their recovery. Health-care workers should take special note of women's reports of pain, since pain may be due to uterine perforation (which may require observation or laparotomy for treatment) or acute haematometra (blood filling the uterus, which can be treated by re-aspiration of the uterine cavity). Thus, particularly with late abortions, it is important to confirm manually the size of the

uterus through the abdominal wall. In the absence of complications, most women can leave the health-care facility as soon as they feel able and their vital signs are normal (*19*). After abortions performed later in pregnancy, and after heavy sedation or general anaesthesia, recovery periods may be longer and women may require closer observation.

After a surgical abortion, women may experience light menstrual-like bleeding or spotting for several weeks. Women should be informed that bleeding similar to or heavier than a heavy menstrual period might be expected with medical methods of abortion. Symptoms that warrant clinical attention include excessive bleeding, fever lasting more than one day, and worsening pelvic pain, or, rarely, signs of ongoing pregnancy. Nausea, sometimes accompanied by vomiting, generally subsides within 24 hours after surgical abortion. Staff should advise women to expect cramping, which they can usually alleviate sufficiently with non-prescription non-steroidal anti-inflammatory drugs, such as ibuprofen. Information on recognizing complications and where and how to seek help for them should be made available in pictorial form for women who cannot read.

After first-trimester abortion, most women can return to their usual activities and responsibilities within hours or days (*19*). Women undergoing surgical abortion may be offered a follow-up visit with a trained practitioner, within 2 weeks after the procedure. This visit can be an opportunity for providers to talk with women about their experiences, if needed. For example, women having an abortion for medical reasons, or following rape, may need to speak about their sense of loss or ambivalence, or may want additional counselling.

2.3.2 Medical methods of abortion

Due to the high effectiveness of the mifepristone and misoprostol combination for medical abortion up to 9 weeks (63 days) of gestation, there is no need for medical follow-up to confirm completed abortion. Women, however, should be advised to return for follow-up if they are experiencing signs of ongoing pregnancy or for other medical reasons, such as prolonged heavy bleeding or fever. Those who had a medical abortion using a misoprostol-only regimen should return for follow-up for confirmation of complete abortion 7–14 days following misoprostol intake.

Treatment protocols for mifepristone followed by misoprostol used up to 9 weeks of pregnancy that require women to remain under clinical observation for 4–6 hours after taking the misoprostol should have confirmation of an abortion during this time, if possible. Confirmation is generally made by inspecting sanitary pads and bed pans used during the period of observation, for expelled products of conception.

Complete abortion may be confirmed by pelvic examination, pelvic ultrasound or a repeat hCG measurement. If hCG measurements are used, it should be remembered that in some cases low hCG levels can be detectable for up to 4 weeks after successful expulsion. Ultrasound is useful to detect ongoing pregnancy; measuring endometrial thickness, however, is not useful for diagnosing incomplete abortion and may lead to inappropriate surgical interventions (132). Women who continue to have symptoms of pregnancy or have minimal bleeding are likely to be still pregnant.

Women with failed abortion (the pregnancy is ongoing) should be offered either vacuum aspiration or repeat administration of misoprostol. Available data regarding a potential risk of fetal abnormality after an unsuccessful medical abortion are limited and inconclusive; therefore, it is unnecessary to insist on termination of an exposed pregnancy if the woman wishes to continue it. Women should, nevertheless, be informed that due to the unknown risk to the fetus of abortifacient drugs, follow-up is important (12, 133).

Women with incomplete abortions can generally be observed unless vaginal bleeding is heavy, or they may be offered re-administration of misoprostol or surgical completion of their abortion. In view of the greater risk of haemorrhage and of incomplete abortion associated with procedures undertaken after 12 weeks of pregnancy, all women in these situations should remain under clinical observation until both the fetus and placenta have been expelled. Additionally, medical abortions after 9 weeks' gestation should take place in a health-care facility, although research is ongoing to determine whether home abortion among a subgroup of this gestational age range is safe and appropriate.

References

1. Bartlett LA et al. Risk factors for legal induced abortion-related mortality in the United States. *Obstetrics and Gynecology*, 2004, 103:729–737.

2. Grimes DA, Cates W, Jr. Complications from legally-induced abortion: a review. *Obstetrical and Gynecological Survey*, 1979, 34(3):177–191.

3. Royal College of Obstetricians and Gynaecologists. *The care of women requesting induced abortion.* Evidence-based guideline no. 7. London, RCOG Press, 2004.

4. Kulier R et al. Medical methods for first trimester abortion. *Cochrane Database of Systematic Reviews*, 2011, (1):CD002855.

5. Kulier R, Kapp N. Comprehensive analysis of the use of pre-procedure ultrasound for first- and second-trimester abortion. *Contraception*, 2010, 83:30–33.

6. Laing FD, Frates MC. Ultrasound evaluation during the first trimester of pregnancy. In: Callen P, ed. *Ultrasonography in obstetrics and gynecology*, 4th ed. Philadelphia, WB Saunders, 2010:118–119.

7. Penney GC et al. A randomised comparison of strategies for reducing infective complications of induced abortion. *British Journal of Obstetrics and Gynaecology*, 1998, 105:599–604.

8. Low N et al. Perioperative antibiotics to prevent infection after first-trimester abortion. *Cochrane Database of Systematic Reviews*, 2012, (3):CD005217.

9. Sawaya GF et al. Antibiotics at the time of induced abortion: the case for universal prophylaxis based on a metaanalysis. *Obstetrics and Gynecology*, 1996, 87:884–890.

10. Shannon C et al. Infection after medical abortion: a review of the literature. *Contraception*, 2004, 70:183–190.

11. *Managing the complications of pregnancy and childbirth: a guide for midwives and doctors*, 2nd ed. Geneva, World Health Organization, 2003.

12. *Frequently asked clinical questions about medical abortion*. Geneva, World Health Organization, 2006.

13. Majhi AK et al. Ectopic pregnancy-an analysis of 180 cases. *Journal of the Indian Medical Association*, 2007, 105:308–312.

14. Barnhart KT et al. Risk factors for ectopic pregnancy in women with symptomatic first-trimester pregnancies. *Fertility and Sterility*, 2006, 86:36–43.

15. Finn R et al. Experimental studies on prevention of Rh haemolytic disease. *British Medical Journal*, 1961, 1(523):1486–1490.

16. Naik K et al. The incidence of fetomaternal haemorrhage following elective termination of first-trimester pregnancy. *European Journal of Obstetrics Gynecology and Reproductive Biology*, 1988, 27:355–357.

17. Fiala C, Fux M, Gemzell DK. Rh-prophylaxis in early abortion. *Acta Obstetrica et Gynecologica Scandinavica*, 2003, 82:892–903.

18. Urquhart DR, Templeton A. Reduced risk of iso-immunisation in medical abortion. *Lancet*, 1990, 335:914.

19. *Safe abortion: technical and policy guidance for health systems*. Geneva, World Health Organization, 2003.

20. Baker A, Beresford T. Informed consent, patient education and counseling. In: Paul M et al. eds. *Management of unintended and abnormal pregnancy: comprehensive abortion care*. Hoboken, NJ, Wiley-Blackwell, 2009:48–62.

21. Henshaw RC et al. Comparison of medical abortion with surgical vacuum aspiration: women's preferences and acceptability of treatment. *British Medical Journal*, 1993, 307:714–717.

22. Slade P et al. A comparison of medical and surgical termination of pregnancy: choice, emotional impact and satisfaction with care. *British Journal of Obstetrics and Gynaecology*, 1998, 105:1288–1295.

23. Honkanen H, von Hertzen H. Users' perspectives on medical abortion in Finland. *Contraception*, 2002, 65:419–423.

24. Winikoff B et al. Safety, efficacy, and acceptability of medical abortion in China, Cuba, and India: a comparative trial of mifepristone–misoprostol versus surgical abortion. *American Journal of Obstetrics and Gynecology*, 1997, 176:431–437.

25. Honkanen H et al., WHO Research Group on Post-Ovulatory Methods for Fertility Regulation. WHO multinational study of three misoprostol regimens after mifepristone for early medical abortion. *British Journal of Obstetrics and Gynaecology*, 2004, 111:715–725.

26. Cameron IT, Baird DT. The return to ovulation following early abortion – a comparison between vacuum aspiration and prostaglandin. *Acta Endocrinologica*, 1988, 118:161–167.

27. Hamoda H et al. A randomised controlled trial of mifepristone in combination with misoprostol administered sublingually or vaginally for medical abortion up to 13 weeks of gestation. *British Journal of Obstetrics and Gynaecology*, 2005, 112(8):1102–1108.

28. Tang OS et al. Pilot study on the use of repeated doses of sublingual misoprostol in termination of pregnancy up to 12 weeks gestation: efficacy and acceptability. *Human Reproduction,* 2002, 17:654–658.

29. Kapp N et al. Cervical preparation for first trimester surgical abortion. *Cochrane Database of Systematic Reviews*, 2010, (2):CD007207.

30. Newmann SJ et al. Cervical preparation for second trimester dilation and evacuation. *Cochrane Database of Systematic Reviews*, 2010, (8):CD007310.

31. Grimes DA, Schulz KF, Cates WJ. Prevention of uterine perforation during currettage abortion. *Journal of the American Medical Association*, 1984, 251:2108–2112.

32. Schulz KF, Grimes DA, Cates W. Measures to prevent cervical injury during suction curettage abortion. *Lancet*, 1983, 1(8335):1182–1185.

33. Borgatta L, Kapp N. Clinical guidelines. Labor induction abortion in the second trimester. *Contraception*, 2011, 84(1):4–18.

34. World Health Organization, Task Force on Postovulatory Methods for Fertility Regulation. *Cervical ripening with mifepristone (RU 486) in late first trimester abortion*. Geneva, World Health Organization, 1994 (Report No. 50).

35. Smith G et al. Pain of first trimester abortion: its quantification and relations with other variables. *American Journal of Obstetrics and Gynecology*, 1979, 133:489–498.

36. Belanger E, Melzack R, Lauzon P. Pain of first-trimester abortion: a study of psychosocial and medical predictors. *Pain*, 1989, 36:339–350.

37. Renner RM et al. Pain control in first trimester surgical abortion. *Cochrane Database of Systematic Reviews*, 2009;(2):CD006712.

38. Borgatta L, Nickinovich D. Pain during early abortion. *Journal of Reproductive Medicine*, 1997, 42:287–293.

39. Solo J. Easing the pain: pain management in the treatment of incomplete abortion. *Reproductive Health Matters*, 2000, 8:45–51.

40. Faymonville ME et al. Psychological approaches during conscious sedation. Hypnosis versus stress reducing strategies: a prospective randomized study. *Pain*, 1997, 73:361–367.

41. Marc I et al. The use of hypnosis to improve pain management during voluntary interruption of pregnancy: an open randomized preliminary study. *Contraception*, 2007, 75:52–58.

42. Suprapto K, Reed S. Naproxen sodium for pain relief in first-trimester abortion. *American Journal of Obstetrics and Gynecology*, 1984, 150:1000–1001.

43. Matambo J, Moodley J, Chigumadzi P. Analgesia for termination of pregnancy. *South African Medical Journal*, 1999, 89:816.

44. Cade L, Ashley J. Prophylactic paracetamol for analgesia after vaginal termination of pregnancy. *Anaesthesia and Intensive Care*, 1993, 21:93–96.

45. Hein A, Jakobsson J, Ryberg G. Paracetamol 1 g given rectally at the end of minor gynaecological surgery is not efficacious in reducing postoperative pain. *Acta Anaesthesiologica Scandinavica*, 1999, 43:248–251.

46. Dahl V, Fjellanger F, Raeder JC. No effect of pre-operative paracetamol and codeine suppositories for pain after termination of pregnancies in general anaesthesia. *European Journal of Pain*, 2000, 4:211–215.

47. Jackson E, Kapp N. Pain control in first and second trimester medical termination of pregnancy: a systematic review. *Contraception*, 2011, 83:116–126.

48. Lawson HW et al. Abortion mortality, United States, 1972 through 1987. *American Journal of Obstetrics and Gynecology*, 1994, 171:1365–1372.

49. Mackay H, Schulz KF, Grimes D. Safety of local versus general anaesthesia for second trimester dilation and evacuation abortion. *Obstetrics and Gynecology*, 1985, 66:661–665.

50. Osborn JF et al. General-anesthesia, a risk factor for complication following induced-abortion. *European Journal of Epidemiology*, 1990, 6:416–422.

51. Drey E et al. Safety of intra-amniotic digoxim administration before late second-trimester abortion by dilation and evacuation. *American Journal of Obstetrics and Gynecology*, 2000, 182:1063–1066.

52. Lalitkumar S et al. Mid-trimester induced abortion: a review. *Human Reproduction Update*, 2007, 13:37–52.

53. Hammond C. Recent advances in second-trimester abortion: an evidence-based review. *American Journal of Obstetrics and Gynecology*, 2009, 200:347–356.

54. Nucatola D, Roth N, Gatter M. A randomized pilot study on the effectiveness and side-effect profiles of two doses of digoxin as fetocide when administered intraamniotically or intrafetally prior to second-trimester surgical abortion. *Contraception*, 2010, 81:67–74.

55. Greenslade F et al. Summary of clinical and programmatic experience with manual vacuum aspiration. *IPAS Advances in Abortion Care*, 1993, 3:1–4.

56. Niinimaki M et al. Immediate complications after medical compared with surgical termination of pregnancy. *Obstetrics and Gynecology*, 2009, 114:795–804.

57. Kulier R et al. Surgical methods for first trimester termination of pregnancy. *Cochrane Database of Systematic Reviews*, 2009, (4):CD002900.

58. Creinin MD. Randomized comparison of efficacy, acceptability and cost of medical versus surgical abortion. *Contraception*, 2000, 62:117–124.

59. Paul M et al, eds. *Management of unintended and abnormal pregnancy: comprehensive abortion care*. Hoboken, NJ, Wiley-Blackwell, 2009.

60. Hakim-Elahi E, Tovell HM, Burnhill MS. Complications of first-trimester abortion: a report of 170,000 cases. *Obstetrics and Gynecology*, 1990, 76:129–135.

61. Cates W, Grimes DA, Schulz KF. Abortion surveillance at CDC – creating public health light out of political heat. *American Journal of Preventive Medicine*, 2000, 19:12–17.

62. Grimes DA et al. The Joint Program for the Study of Abortion/CDC – a preliminary report. Abortion in the seventies. In: Hern WM, Andrikopoulos B, eds. *Abortion in the seventies: proceedings of the Western Regional Conference on Abortion*. New York, National Abortion Federation, 1977:41–54.

63. Lean T et al. A comparison of D&C and vacuum aspiration for performing first trimester abortion. *International Journal of Gynecology and Obstetrics*, 1976, 14:481–486.

64. Say L et al. Medical versus surgical methods for first trimester termination of pregnancy. *Cochrane Database of Systematic Reviews*, 2005, (1):CD003037.

65. Darney PD, Sweet RL. Routine intraoperative ultrasonography for second trimester abortion reduces incidence of uterine perforation. *Journal of Ultrasound Medicine*, 1989, 8:71–75.

66. Grimes DA, Hulka JF, McCuthen ME. Midtrimester abortion by dilatation and evacuation versus intra-amniotic instillation of prostglandin F2 alpha: a randomized clinical trial. *American Journal of Obstetrics and Gynecology*, 1980, 137:785–790.

67. Grimes DA, Smith MS, Witham AD. Mifepristone and misoprostol versus dilation and evacuation for midtrimester abortion: a pilot randomised controlled trial. *British Journal of Obstetrics and Gynaecology*, 2004, 111(2):148–153.

68. Lohr PA, Hayes JL, Gemzell-Danielsson K. Surgical versus medical methods for second trimester induced abortion. *Cochrane Database of Systematic Reviews*, 2008, (1):CD006714.

69. Ashok PW et al. An effective regimen for early medical abortion: a report of 2000 consecutive cases. *Human Reproduction*, 1998, 13:2962–2965.

70. Trussell J, Ellertson C. Estimating the efficacy of medical abortion. *Contraception*, 1999, 60:119–135.

71. Urquhart DR et al. The efficacy and tolerance of mifepristone and prostaglandin in termination of pregnancy of less than 63 days gestation; UK multicentre study – final results. *Contraception*, 1997, 55:1–5.

72. Swahn ML, Bygdeman M. The effect of the antiprogestin RU 486 on uterine contractility and sensitivity to prostaglandin and oxytocin. *British Journal of Obstetrics and Gynaecology*, 1988, 95:126–134.

73. *WHO model list of essential medicines*, 16th ed. Geneva, World Health Organization, 2010.

74. Sang G, He C, Shao Q. A large-scale introductory trial on termination of early pregnancy by mifepristone in combination with different prostaglandins. *Chinese Journal of Clinical Pharmacology*, 1999, 15:323–329.

75. Creinin MD, Aubeny E. Medical abortion in early pregnancy. In: Paul M et al, eds. *A clinician's guide to medical and surgical abortion*. New York, Churchill Livingstone, 1999:91–106.

76. Elul B et al. Side effects of mifepristone-misoprostol abortion versus surgical abortion – data from a trial in China, Cuba, and India. *Contraception*, 1999, 59:107–114.

77. Ngoc NTN et al. Safety, efficacy and acceptability of mifepristone-misoprostol medical abortion in Vietnam. *International Family Planning Perspectives*, 1999, 25:10–14 and 33.

78. Tran NT et al. Feasibility, efficacy, safety and acceptability of mifepristone-misoprostol for medical abortion in the Democratic People's Republic of Korea. *International Journal of Gynaecology and Obstetrics*, 2010, 109:209–212.

79. *Essential medicines: WHO model list*, 12th ed. Geneva, World Health Organization, 2002.

80. Fjerstad M et al. Rates of serious infection after changes in regimens for medical abortion. *New England Journal of Medicine*, 2009, 361:145–151.

81. World Health Organization, Task Force on Post-ovulatory Methods for Fertility Regulation. Comparison of two doses of mifepristone in combination with misoprostol for early medical abortion: a randomised trial. *British Journal of Obstetrics and Gynaecology*, 2000, 107:524–530.

82. Mckinley C, Thong KJ, Baird DT. The effect of dose of mifepristone and gestation on the efficacy of medical abortion with mifepristone and misoprostol. *Human Reproduction*, 1993, 8:1502–1505.

83. World Health Organization Task Force on Post-ovulatory Methods for Fertility Regulation. Termination of pregnancy with reduced doses of mifepristone. *British Medical Journal*, 1993, 307:532–537.

84. World Health Organization. Pregnancy termination with mifepristone and gemeprost: a multicenter comparison between repeated doses and a single dose of mifepristone. *Fertility and Sterility*, 1991, 56:32–40.

85. World Health Organization Task Force on Post-ovulatory Methods for Fertility Regulation. Lowering the doses of mifepristone and gameprost for early abortion: a randomised controlled trial. *British Journal of Obstetrics and Gynaecology*, 2001, 108:738–742.

86. von Hertzen H et al. Two mifepristone doses and two intervals of misoprostol administration for termination of early pregnancy: a randomised factorial controlled equivalence trial. *British Journal of Obstetrics and Gynaecology*, 2009, 116:381–389.

87. Elrefaey H et al. Induction of abortion with mifepristone (Ru-486) and oral or vaginal misoprostol. *New England Journal of Medicine*, 1995, 332:983–987.

88. Ngo TD et al. *Comparative effectiveness, safety and acceptability of medical abortion at home and in a clinic: a systematic review*. Geneva, World Health Organization, 2011 (Report no. 89).

89. Hajri S et al. Expanding medical abortion in Tunisia: women's experiences from a multi-site expansion study. *Contraception*, 2004, 70:487–491.

90. Breitbart V. Counseling for medical abortion. *American Journal of Obstetrics and Gynecology*, 2000, 183(2 Suppl.):S26–S33.

Clinical care for women undergoing abortion

91. Wildschut H et al. Medical methods for mid-trimester termination of pregnancy. *Cochrane Database of Systematic Reviews*, 2010, (2):CD005216.

92. Ho PC, Chan YF, Lau W. Misoprostol is as effective as gemeprost in termination of second trimester pregnancy when combined with mifepristone: a randomised comparative trial. *Contraception*, 1996, 53:281–283.

93. Gemzell-Danielsson K, Ostlund E. Termination of second trimester pregnancy with mifepristone and gemeprost – the clinical experience of 197 consecutive cases. *Acta Obstetricia et Gynecologica Scandinavica*, 2000, 79:702–706.

94. Tang OS, Thong KJ, Baird DT. Second trimester medical abortion with mifepristone and gemeprost: a review of 956 cases. *Contraception*, 2001, 64:29–32.

95. Bugalho A et al. Termination of pregnancies of <6 weeks gestation with a single dose of 800 µg of vaginal misoprostol. *Contraception*, 2000, 61:47–50.

96. Costa SH, Vessey MP. Misoprostol and illegal abortion in Rio-De-Janeiro, Brazil. *Lancet*, 1993, 341:1258–1261.

97. Faundes A et al. Misoprostol for the termination of pregnancy up to 12 completed weeks of pregnancy. *International Journal of Gynaecology and Obstetrics*, 2007, 99(Suppl. 2):S172–S177.

98. Ho PC et al. Misoprostol for the termination of pregnancy with a live fetus at 13 to 26 weeks. *International Journal of Gynaecology and Obstetrics*, 2007, 99(Suppl. 2):S178–S181.

99. Thong KJ, Robertson AJ, Baird DT. A retrospective study of 932 second trimester terminations using gemeprost (16,16 dimethyl-trans delta 2 PGE1 methyl ester). *Prostaglandins*, 1992, 44:65–74.

100. UNDP/UNFPA/WHO/World Bank Special Programme of Research, Development and Research Training in Human Reproduction. Methotrexate for the termination of early pregnancy: a toxicology review. *Reproductive Health Matters*, 1997, 9:162–166.

101. Powell HR, Ekert H. Methotrexate-induced congenital malformations. *Medical Journal of Australia*,1971, 2:1076–1077.

102. Diniz E et al. Efietos sobre o concepto do metotrexato (ametopterina) administrado à mae. Apresentaçao de caso. *Revista do Hospital das Clinicas, Faculdade de Medicine à Universidade de Sao Paulo*, 1978, 33:286–290.

103. Feldkamp M, Carey JC. Clinical teratology counseling and consultation case-report – low-dose methotrexate exposure in the early weeks of pregnancy. *Teratology*, 1993, 47:533–539.

104. *Clinical management of abortion complications: a practical guide*. Geneva, World Health Organization, 1994.

105. Tuncalp O, Gulmezoglu AM, Souza J. Surgical procedures to evacuate incomplete miscarriage. *Cochrane Database of Systematic Reviews*, 2010, (1):CD001993.

106. Neilson JP et al. Medical treatments for incomplete miscarriage (less than 24 weeks). *Cochrane Database of Systematic Reviews*, 2010, (1):CD007223.

107. Diop A et al. Two routes of administration for misoprostol in the treatment of incomplete abortion: a randomized clinical trial. *Contraception*, 2009, 79:456–462.

108. Tang OS et al. Pharmacokinetics of repeated doses of misoprostol. *Human Reproduction*, 2009, 24:1862–1869.

109. *FDA public health advisory; sepsis and medical abortion.* Silver Spring, MD, US Food and Drug Administration, 2010.

110. Ho CS et al. Undiagnosed cases of fatal Clostridium-associated toxic shock in Californian women of childbearing age. *American Journal of Obstetrics and Gynecology*, 2009, 201:459–457.

111. Kaali SG, Szigetvari IA, Bartfai GS. The frequency and management of uterine perforations during 1st-trimester abortions. *American Journal of Obstetrics and Gynecology*, 1989, 161:406–408.

112. Goyal V. Uterine rupture in second-trimester misoprostol-induced abortion after cesarean delivery: a systematic review. *Obstetrics and Gynecology*, 2009, 113:1117–1123.

113. *Medical methods for termination of pregnancy.* WHO Technical Report Series 871. Geneva, World Health Organization, 1997.

114. Atrash HK, Hogue CJ. The effect of pregnancy termination on future reproduction. *Baillières Clinical Obstetrics and Gynaecology*, 1990, 4:391–405.

115. Virk J, Zhang J, Olsen J. Medical abortion and the risk of subsequent adverse pregnancy outcomes. *New England Journal of Medicine*, 2007, 357:648–653.

116. Cates W Jr, Grimes DA, Schulz KF. The public health impact of legal abortion: 30 years later. *Perspectives on Sexual and Reproductive Health*, 2003, 35:25–28.

117. Rowland Hogue CJ et al. Answering questions about long-term outcomes. In Paul M et al., eds. *Management of unintended and abnormal pregnancy: comprehensive abortion care.* Hoboken, NJ, Wiley-Blackwell, 2009:252–263.

118. Lurie S et al. The influence of midtrimester termination of pregnancy on subsequent fertility: four to five years follow-up. *Contraception*, 1994, 50:239–241.

119. Beral V et al. Breast cancer and abortion: collaborative reanalysis of data from 53 epidemiological studies, including 83 000 women with breast cancer from 3.6 countries. *Lancet*, 2004, 363:1007–1016.

120. Melbye M et al. Induced abortion and the risk of breast cancer. *New England Journal of Medicine*, 1997, 336:81–85.

121. Dagg PKB. The psychological sequelae of therapeutic-abortion – denied and completed. *American Journal of Psychiatry*, 1991, 148:578–585.

122. Major B et al. Abortion and mental health evaluating the evidence. *American Psychologist*, 2009, 64:863–890.

123. World Health Organization. Standard precautions in health care. *WHO Infection Control*, October 2007, Epidemic and Pandemic Alert and Response (http://www.who.int/csr/resources/publications/EPR_AM2_E7.pdf, accessed 1 September 2011).

124. *WHO guidelines on hand hygiene and health care. First global patient safety challenge, clean care is safer care.* Geneva, World Health Organization, 2009 (http://whqlibdoc.who.int/publications/2009/9789241597906_eng.pdf, accessed 1 September 2011).

125. Sopwith W, Hart T, Garner P. Preventing infection from reusable medical equipment: a systematic review. *BMC Infectious Diseases*, 2002, 2:4.

126. Tietjen L, Bossemeyer D, McIntosh N. *Infection prevention: guidelines for healthcare facilities with limited resources.* Baltimore, MD, Jhpiego, 2003 (http://pdf.usaid.gov/pdf_docs/PNACT433.pdf, accessed 1 September 2011).

127. World Health Organization and Johns Hopkins Blomberg School of Public Health/Center for Communication Programs (CCP) IP. *Family planning: a global handbook for providers.* Baltimore and Geneva, CCP and WHO, 2008.

128. Goodman S et al. A. Impact of immediate postabortal insertion of intrauterine contraception on repeat abortion. *Contraception*, 2008, 78:143–148.

129. Reeves MF, Smith KJ, Creinin MD. Contraceptive effectiveness of immediate compared with delayed insertion of intrauterine devices after abortion: a decision analysis. *Obstetrics and Gynecology*, 2007, 109:1286–1294.

130. Roberts H, Silva M, Xu S. Post abortion contraception and its effect on repeat abortions in Auckland, New Zealand. *Contraception*, 2010, 82:260–265.

131. Stanwood NL, Grimes DA, Schulz KF. Insertion of an intrauterine contraceptive device after induced or spontaneous abortion: a review of the evidence. *British Journal of Obstetrics and Gynaecology*, 2001, 108:1168–1173.

132. Reeves MF et al. Endometrial thickness following medical abortion is not predictive of subsequent surgical intervention. *Ultrasound in Obstetrics and Gynecology*, 2009, 34:104–109.

133. Sitruk-Ware R, Davey A, Sakiz E. Fetal malformation and failed medical termination of pregnancy. *Lancet*, 1998, 352:323.

Chapter 3

CHAPTER 3
Planning and managing safe abortion care

Summary

Planning and managing safe, legal abortion care requires consideration of a number of health system issues. These issues apply whether services are public, private or not-for-profit. In most cases, minor modifications of existing facilities, acquisition of minimal additional equipment and medications, and/or provision of basic training can facilitate service provision where none previously existed, or can improve the quality, safety, efficiency and capacity of existing services. Establishing and/or strengthening existing services should be based on careful planning encompassing the following principles and recommendations, which have been generated from reviews of the relevant scientific literature and on recent World Health Organization (WHO) consultative processes (indicated by links to online publications).

- *Establishment of national standards and guidelines* facilitating access to and provision of safe abortion care to the full extent of the law. Standards and guidelines should cover: types of abortion service, where and by whom they can be provided; essential equipment, instruments, medications, supplies and facility capabilities; referral mechanisms; respect for women's informed decision-making, autonomy, confidentiality and privacy, with attention to the special needs of adolescents; special provisions for women who have suffered rape; and conscientious objection by health-care providers.

- *Ensuring health-care provider skills and performance* through: training; supportive and facilitative supervision; monitoring, evaluation, and other quality-improvement processes. Training should be competency based and address health-care provider attitudes and ethical issues related to the provision of safe, induced abortion (http://whqlibdoc.who.int/publications/2011/9789241501002_eng.pdf). Monitoring and evaluation include the collection of routine service statistics and safe abortion indicators, the use of checklists, periodic special studies, and feedback mechanisms to ensure continuous quality improvement (http://www.who.int/reproductivehealth/publications/monitoring/924156315x/en/index.html).

- *Financing*: health-service budgets should include the costs of staff, training programmes, equipment, medications, supplies and capital costs. Consideration also needs to be given to making services affordable to women who need them. The costs of adding safe abortion services to existing health services are likely to be modest, relative to the costs to the health system of unsafe abortion and to gains for women's health (http://screening.iarc.fr/doc/policybrief1.pdf).

- *A systematic approach to policy and programme development*: this means planning and implementing policies and programmes with the end result – promoting women's health and their human rights – in mind. It involves assessing the current situation; introducing interventions and testing their feasibility, acceptability and effectiveness on a small scale; and then scaling-up successful interventions so that the benefits can have broader impacts on health-system performance and the health and well-being of women, their families and communities (http://www.who.int/reproductivehealth/publications/strategic_approach/9789241500319/en/index.html).

3.1 Introduction

This chapter sets out considerations for establishing and/or strengthening safe abortion care. It highlights the key components of safe abortion care as well as the process of putting policies, programmes and services in place, including issues such as assessment of needs and priorities, introducing interventions on a small scale, and scaling-up successful interventions for broader impact.

Policy-makers and health-care managers working to provide reproductive health services should always ensure that safe abortion care is readily accessible and available to the full extent of the law. Women in all countries have induced abortions. Where legal services are readily accessible and available, those abortions are generally safe; where access and availability of legal services are highly restricted, they tend to be unsafe (1, 2). Abortion laws and services should protect the health and human rights of all women, including adolescents. They should not create situations that lead women and adolescents to seek unsafe abortion. Indeed, most countries have one or more legal indications for the provision of safe abortion. However, in countries with highly restrictive laws on induced abortion, services may be largely limited to the treatment of complications from unsafe abortion. Such treatment is often referred to as "post-abortion care". Emergency treatment of abortion complications is essential to reduce deaths and injuries from unsafe abortion but it cannot replace the protection of women's health and their human rights afforded by safe, legal induced abortion.

3.2 Constellation of services

Abortion services should be integrated into the health system, either as public services or through publicly funded, non-profit services, to acknowledge their status as legitimate health services and to protect against stigmatization and discrimination of women and health-care providers.

Constellation of services should always involve, at a minimum:

- medically accurate information about abortion in a form the woman can understand and recall, and non-directive counselling if requested by the woman to facilitate informed decision-making;

- abortion services delivered without delay;

- timely treatment for abortion complications, including complications from unsafe abortion;

- contraceptive information, services and referrals, to help prevent repeat unintended pregnancy and reduce the need for another abortion.

Access to safe abortion depends not only on the availability of services, but also on the manner in which they are delivered and the treatment of women within the clinical context. Services should be delivered in a way that respects a woman's dignity, guarantees her right to privacy and is sensitive to her needs and perspectives. Attention should be given to the special needs of the poor, adolescents, and other vulnerable and marginalized women.

3.3 Evidence-based standards and guidelines

In many countries, evidence-based standards and guidelines for abortion service delivery, including treatment of abortion complications, do not exist. Standards for abortion care refer to the underlying principles and essential requirements for providing equitable access to, and adequate quality of, lawful abortion services. Guidelines for abortion care are evidence-based recommendations for the delivery of safe abortion care. In countries where standards and guidelines already exist, routine review and updates ensure that they continue to promote women's physical, mental, and social well-being and reflect new evidence of best practices. Standards and guidelines should be developed and updated with the intent of eliminating barriers to obtaining the highest attainable standard of sexual and reproductive health.

3.3.1 Types of abortion services, where and by whom they can be provided

The availability of facilities and trained providers within reach of the entire population is essential to ensuring access to safe abortion services. Regulation of providers and facilities should be based on evidence of best practices and be aimed at ensuring safety, good quality and accessibility of services. Abortion facilities within both the public and private sectors should be available at all levels of the health system, with appropriate referral mechanisms between facilities.

Abortion care can be safely provided by any properly trained health-care provider, including midlevel (i.e. non-physician) providers (3–5, 6). The term "midlevel providers" in the context of this document refers to a range of non-physician clinicians (e.g. midwives, nurse practitioners, clinical officers, physician assistants, family welfare visitors, and others) who are trained to provide basic clinical procedures related to reproductive health, including bimanual pelvic examination to determine age of pregnancy and positioning of the uterus, uterine sounding and other transcervical procedures, and who can be trained to provide safe abortion care.

Abortion care provided at the primary-care level and through outpatient services in higher-level settings is safe, and minimizes costs while maximizing the convenience and timeliness of care for the woman (7). Where capacity to provide good-quality abortion services at the primary level does not yet exist, referral to services at higher levels is essential (see Box 3.1). Allowing home use of misoprostol following provision of mifepristone at the health-care facility can further improve the privacy, convenience and acceptability of services, without compromising on safety (8–10). Inpatient abortion care should be reserved for the management of medical abortion for pregnancies of gestational age over 9 weeks (63 days) and management of severe abortion complications (see Chapter 2).

3.3.1.1 Community level

Community-based health-care workers can play an important role in helping women avoid unintended pregnancy, through providing contraceptive information, counselling and methods, and informing them about the risks of unsafe abortion (11). They can also inform women about where to obtain a pregnancy test and how to obtain safe, legal abortion care, and they can refer women with complications from unsafe abortion for emergency care. Chemists/pharmacists, like community health-care workers, can help women avoid unintended pregnancy through provision of accurate contraceptive information and methods. They can also provide pregnancy tests and referral to safe abortion services.

BOX 3.1

Types of service suitable to each level of the health system

Community level:

- public health education/information on reproductive health, including contraception and abortion;
- community-based distribution of appropriate methods of contraception;
- all health-care workers trained to provide information on, and referral to, pregnancy-detection and safe, legal abortion services;
- all health-care workers trained to recognize abortion complications and promptly refer women for treatment;
- transportation to services for management of complications of abortion;
- all health-care workers (and other key community professionals such as police or teachers) trained to recognize signs of rape and to provide referral to health-care or other social services.

Primary-care facility level:

- all elements of care mentioned for the community level;
- all health-care workers providing reproductive health services trained to provide counselling on contraception, unintended pregnancy and abortion;
- a broad range of contraceptive methods, including IUDs, implants, and injectables;
- vacuum aspiration (manual or electric) for pregnancies of gestational age up to 12–14 weeks (see Chapter 2);
- medical methods of abortion for pregnancies of gestational age up to 9 weeks, or up to 12 weeks if the woman can stay in the facility until the abortion is complete (see Chapter 2);
- clinical stabilization, provision of antibiotics, and uterine evacuation for women with complications of abortion;
- vacuum aspiration or treatment with misoprostol for incomplete abortion;
- prompt referral for women needing services for abortion or for management of abortion complications that cannot be provided on-site.

Referral hospitals:

- all elements of abortion care mentioned for the primary-care level;
- provision of sterilization in addition to other contraceptive methods;
- abortion services for all circumstances and stages of pregnancy, as permitted by law;
- management of all abortion complications;
- information and outreach programmes covering the full catchment area;
- training of all relevant cadres of health-care professionals in abortion provision.

3.3.1.2 Primary-care facility level

Both vacuum aspiration and medical abortion can be provided at the primary-care level on an outpatient basis and do not require advanced technical knowledge or skills, expensive equipment such as ultrasound, or a full complement of hospital staff (e.g. anaesthesiologist) (*12*). Primary health-care staff are likely to include nurses, midwives, health-care assistants and, in some contexts, physicians. Health-care personnel with the skills to perform a bimanual pelvic examination to diagnose and date a pregnancy, and to perform a transcervical procedure such as intrauterine device (IUD) insertion, can be trained to perform vacuum aspiration (*5, 6, 13–15*). Where medical methods of abortion are registered and available, midlevel health-care providers can also administer and supervise abortion services (*3, 16, 17*). For both vacuum aspiration and medical abortion, procedures for referral to higher-level care should be in place (*12*).

3.3.1.3 Referral hospitals

Referral hospitals should have the staff and capacity to perform abortions in all circumstances permitted by law and to manage all abortion complications.

3.3.2 Methods of abortion

Respect for a woman's choice among different safe and effective methods of abortion is an important value in health-service delivery. Although the choice of methods will reflect health-system capability, even the most resource-constrained health systems should be able to provide medical methods and manual vacuum aspiration. Where a choice of methods cannot be offered, at least one recommended method should always be available. Vacuum aspiration and medical methods should also be widely available to treat women with complications from spontaneous as well as unsafe abortion.

3.3.3 Certification and licensing of health-care professionals and facilities

Where certification of abortion providers is required, it should ensure that health-care providers meet the criteria for provision of abortion care according to national standards, and it should not create barriers to accessing legal services. The certification and licensing of abortion-care services should be the same as for other medical procedures and should not be a barrier to the availability and provision of abortion care.

Licensing criteria, where required, should not impose excessive requirements for infrastructure, equipment, or staff that are not essential to the provision of safe services. Facility licensing criteria should clearly differentiate between requirements at primary-care level versus requirements at referral levels, in order to facilitate, rather than restrict, access to care. Licensing criteria should be the same for both the public and private sectors and not-for-profit facilities.

3.3.4 Referral mechanisms

As with all health interventions, well-functioning referral systems are essential for the provision of safe abortion care. Timely referrals to appropriate facilities reduce delays in seeking care, enhance safety, and can mitigate the severity of abortion complications (*12*).

3.3.5 Respect for women's informed and voluntary decision-making, autonomy, confidentiality and privacy, with attention to adolescents and women with special needs

Within the framework of national abortion laws, norms and standards should include protections for informed and voluntary decision-making, autonomy in decision-making, non-discrimination, and confidentiality and privacy for all women, including adolescents (*18*). These human rights are enshrined in international and regional human rights treaties, as well as in national constitutions and laws.

3.3.5.1 Informed and voluntary decision-making

Depending upon the context and her individual situation, a woman trying to resolve the decision about an unintended pregnancy may feel vulnerable. She needs to be treated with respect and understanding and to be provided with information in a way that she can understand so that she can make a decision free of inducement, coercion or discrimination. Health-care providers should be trained to support women's informed and voluntary decision-making. They should also be aware of situations in which a woman may be coerced into having an abortion against her will (e.g. based on her health status, such as living with HIV). Extra attention is needed in such cases, to ensure that the woman is fully informed and makes a free decision.

3.3.5.2 Third-party authorization

A woman seeking an abortion is an autonomous adult. Autonomy means that mentally competent adults do not require the authorization of any third party, such as a husband, partner, parent or guardian, to access a health service. Therefore, health-care providers should not impose a requirement of third-party authorization unless required by law and related regulations.

Adolescents may be deterred from going to needed health services if they think they will be required to get permission from their parents or guardians, which increases the likelihood of them going to clandestine abortion providers. Health-care providers should therefore be trained to inform, counsel and treat adolescents according to their evolving capacities to understand the treatment and care options being offered, and not according to an arbitrary age cut-off

(*19*). Health-care workers should support minors to identify what is in their best interests, including consulting parents or other trusted adults about their pregnancy, without bias, discrimination or coercion.

3.3.5.3 Protection of persons with special needs

Depending upon the context, unmarried women, adolescents, those living in extreme poverty, women from ethnic minorities, refugees and other displaced persons, women with disabilities, and those facing violence in the home, may be vulnerable to inequitable access to safe abortion services. Abortion-service providers should ensure that all women are treated without discrimination and with respect.

Stigma and discrimination associated with physical and mental disabilities, and health status such as living with HIV, are widespread and may be used as a reason to coerce women into having an abortion. Coercion violates women's rights to informed consent and dignity, and should not be tolerated (*20*). Thus, health-care providers have a human rights obligation to ensure that women are not subject to coercion and that they receive the necessary psychological, social and health services to support their choice.

3.3.5.4 Confidentiality and privacy

The fear that confidentiality will not be maintained deters many women – particularly adolescents and unmarried women – from seeking safe, legal abortion services, and may drive them to clandestine, unsafe abortion providers, or to self-induce abortion. Confidentiality is a key principle of medical ethics and an aspect of the right to privacy (*21*) and must be guaranteed. Health-care providers therefore have a duty to protect medical information against unauthorized disclosures, and to ensure that women who do authorize release of their confidential information to others do so freely and on the basis of clear information. Adolescents deemed mature enough to receive counselling without the presence of a parent or other person are entitled to privacy, and may request confidential services and treatment (see Section 3.3.5.2).

Health-service managers should ensure that facilities provide privacy for conversations between women and providers, as well as for actual services. For example, procedure rooms should be partitioned for visual and auditory privacy, and only facility staff required for the induced abortion should be present. There should be a private place for undressing, curtained windows, and cloth or paper drapes to cover the woman during the procedure.

3.3.5.5 Special provisions for women who have suffered rape

Women who are pregnant as a result of rape have a special need for sensitive treatment, and all levels of the health system should be able to offer appropriate care and support. Standards and guidelines for provision of abortion in such cases should be elaborated, and appropriate training given to health-care providers and police. Such standards should not impose unnecessary administrative or judicial procedures such as requiring women to press charges or to identify the rapist (22). The standards should ideally be part of comprehensive standards and guidelines for the overall management of survivors of rape, covering physical and psychological care, emergency contraception, post-exposure prophylaxis for HIV prevention, treatment for sexually transmitted infections (STIs) and injuries, collection of forensic evidence, and counselling and follow-up care (20).

3.3.6 Conscientious objection by health-care providers

Health-care professionals sometimes exempt themselves from abortion care on the basis of conscientious objection to the procedure, while not referring the woman to an abortion provider. Individual health-care providers have a right to conscientious objection to providing abortion, but that right does not entitle them to impede or deny access to lawful abortion services because it delays care for women, putting their health and life at risk. In such cases, health-care providers must refer the woman to a willing and trained provider in the same, or another easily accessible health-care facility, in accordance with national law. Where referral is not possible, the health-care professional who objects, must provide safe abortion to save the woman's life and to prevent serious injury to her health. Women who present with complications from an unsafe or illegal abortion must be treated urgently and respectfully, as any other emergency patient, without punitive, prejudiced or biased behaviours (see also Chapter 4).

3.4 Equipping facilities and training health-care providers

The provision of safe abortion care requires properly equipped facilities and well-trained health-care providers. Public health authorities have a responsibility to ensure that systems are in place for continuous and timely procurement and distribution of all medical equipment, drugs, contraceptives and supplies necessary for the safe delivery of services. In addition, health-care providers require appropriate pre-service and in-service training, based on routinely updated guidelines for safe abortion care.

3.4.1 Preparing and equipping facilities

Abortion facilities must be well prepared and equipped to provide safe care. Supportive services, such as commodity procurement, logistics supply chain functioning, and financing mechanisms, are as important as training providers for introducing new

Table 3.1 Drugs, supplies and equipment for safe abortion care

Procedural step	Drugs and supplies	Equipment
Clinical assessment Surgical abortion procedure (equipment for dilatation and evacuation (D&E) highlighted in **bold font**)	• Clean examination gloves • Clean water • Detergent or soap • Cervical preparation agent (e.g. misoprostol tablets, osmotic dilators, mifepristone) • Pain medications, such as analgesics and anxiolytics • Gloves • Gown, face protection • Needles (22 gauge spinal for paracervical block and 21 gauge for drug administration) • Syringes (5, 10 and 20 ml) • Lidocaine for paracervical block • Gauze sponges or cotton balls • Antiseptic solution (non-alcohol based) to prepare the cervix • Instrument-soaking solution • Sterilization or high-level disinfection solutions and materials • Silicone for lubricating syringes	• Blood pressure equipment • Stethoscope • Speculum **(wide mouth to increase exposure of the cervix and short to avoid pushing the cervix away, or a Sims speculum if an assistant is available)** • Tenaculum **(atraumatic tenaculum)** • Tapered dilators up to 37 mm **(up to 51 mm)** or equivalent circumference • Electric vacuum aspirator **(with 14 or 16 mm cannulae)** or MVA aspirator and cannulae up to 12 mm • **Bierer uterine evacuation forceps (large and small)** • **Sopher uterine evacuation forceps (small)** • **Large, postpartum flexible curette** • Sponge (ring) forceps • Stainless steel bowl for prepping solution • Instrument tray • Clear glass dish for tissue inspection • Strainer (metal, glass or gauze)
Medical abortion	• Mifepristone • Misoprostol • Pain medications	• Private area with chairs separate from antenatal or labour care, for women who wait in clinic for expulsion • Adequate toilet facilities
Recovery	• Sanitary napkins or cotton wool • Analgesics • Antibiotics • Information on post-procedure self-care • Post-abortion contraceptive methods and information, and/or referral	• Blood pressure equipment • Stethoscope
In case of complications	• Appropriate antagonists to medications used for pain • Uterotonics (oxytocin, misoprostol or ergometrine) • IV (intravenous) line and fluids (saline, sodium lactate, glucose) • Clear referral mechanisms to higher-level facility, when needed	• Oxygen and Ambu bag • On-site access to an ultrasound machine (optional) • Long needle-driver and suture • Scissors • Uterine packing

services. Where services already exist, infrastructural upgrades can facilitate more efficient patient flow and increase privacy and user satisfaction, while introducing updated methods, such as vacuum aspiration and medical abortion, can improve safety and reduce costs (23, 24).

3.4.1.1 Essential equipment, medications and supplies

Most of the equipment, medications, and supplies needed to provide vacuum aspiration (manual and electric) and medical methods of abortion (see Table 3.1) are the same as those needed for other gynaecological services.

The shift towards using vacuum aspiration with plastic cannulae depends upon official approval and local availability of the instruments. In settings where manual vacuum aspiration (MVA) instruments are not approved medical devices, efforts will be needed to add them to the government's standard equipment list.

These instruments and medications should be routinely included in the planning, budgeting, procurement, distribution and management systems. Criteria for determining what instruments to use include: quality, durability, cost, and system capacity to ensure consistent availability and maintenance over time. As with any other drug, mifepristone and misoprostol for medical abortion should be sourced from manufacturers that adhere to good manufacturing practice (GMP).

Instruments for MVA are made for either single or multiple use. In contexts where instruments will be reused, it is essential to purchase those that can withstand multiple use, cleaning and high-level disinfection or sterilization, as well as to ensure supplies for such disinfection/sterilization. Single-use instruments must be carefully disposed of to avoid health risks to providers and the community. Reusable equipment saves costs, but rigorous cleaning and disinfection procedures must be followed (see Chapter 2).

3.4.1.2 Regulatory requirements for drugs and devices

Each country has specific regulatory requirements for the registration and importation of drugs and medical equipment such as MVA instruments. However, the WHO model list of essential medicines, which has been adapted by many countries as a national essential drugs list, includes combination mifepristone and misoprostol for medical abortion, misoprostol alone for treatment of incomplete abortion and miscarriage, non-narcotic analgesics such as nonsteroidal anti-inflammatory agents (e.g. ibuprofen), tranquillizers (e.g. diazepam) and local anaesthetics (e.g. lidocaine) (25). Inclusion on the national essential drugs list usually means that the drug is registered and available in the country. Where a drug is not registered, some countries will allow importation through the WHO Certification Scheme on the Quality of Pharmaceutical Products Moving in International Commerce (26).

The commodities included in Table 3.1 that are specific to the provision of abortion services should be included in the national medical supplies logistics management programme and be available to healthcare providers that provide abortion services.

3.4.2 Ensuring provider skills and performance

3.4.2.1 Health-care provider skills and training

Health-care providers who perform vacuum aspiration for treatment of incomplete abortion can learn to use the technique for induced abortion, with minimal additional training. All such health-care providers can also be trained to provide medical abortion.

In addition to skills training, participating in values-clarification exercises can help providers differentiate their own personal beliefs and attitudes from the needs of women seeking abortion services (27). Values clarification is an exercise in articulating how personal values influence the way in which providers interact with women seeking abortion. Despite providers' attempts at objectivity, negative and pre-defined beliefs about abortion, and the women who have them, often influence professional judgement and the quality of care (28, 29).

In many contexts, making safe, legal abortion services readily available to all eligible women will require training of midlevel health-care professionals (30–34). Comparative studies have shown no difference in complication rates between women who had first-trimester abortions with MVA performed by midlevel health-care providers and those who had the procedure performed by a physician (6). Skills and performance expectations set out in standards and guidelines should serve as the basis of pre-service training for all appropriate cadres, and abortion-care providers should receive periodic in-service training to ensure they maintain their skills to perform their jobs according to abortion-care standards.

3.4.2.2 Training programmes

As for any other health intervention, abortion training programmes should be competency based and conducted in facilities that have sufficient patient flow to provide all trainees with the requisite practice, including practice in managing abortion complications. In addition, training should address health-care provider attitudes and beliefs about sexual and reproductive health, including induced abortion, safeguarding privacy and confidentiality, treating all women with dignity and respect, and attending the special needs of adolescents, women who have been raped, and those who may be vulnerable for other health or socioeconomic reasons.

Training health-service providers in new or updated clinical procedures can be a powerful tool in changing practices. However, training alone is not sufficient. Trained providers need support following training to put skills into practice, and need to work in an environment that ensures adequate drugs, equipment, remuneration and professional development to support the provision of safe abortion services. They also need supportive and facilitative supervision and oversight to ensure that standards and guidelines are followed. Box 3.2 lists the recommended training content for all health-care professionals providing abortion services.

3.5 Monitoring, evaluation and quality improvement

As with all health services, ensuring good-quality abortion care depends upon effective processes for monitoring, evaluation and quality assurance and improvement. The accurate collection of service statistics and routine monitoring and evaluation at the health-care facility level are a key component of programme management, and feedback based on analysis of these data provides necessary information for improving access and maintaining and improving the quality of services delivered.

BOX 3.2

Recommended training content for abortion-service providers

Background for abortion service delivery:

- legal, regulatory and policy provisions;
- health effects of unsafe abortion;
- ethical responsibility to provide abortion (or to refer women when the health-care professional has conscientious objection to providing abortion) and to treat complications from unsafe abortion;
- national standards and guidelines for abortion care;
- human rights related to safe abortion.

Counselling and provider–patient interaction:

- clarification of health-care provider attitudes and beliefs regarding abortion;
- confidentiality and privacy;
- interpersonal communication and counselling skills;
- information on abortion and contraception;
- issues and risks associated with HIV and other STIs;
- consideration of needs of all women, including adolescents, poor women, women from ethnic minorities, displaced women and refugees, women with disabilities, survivors of rape, women living with HIV or other STIs;
- recognition of signs that the woman has been subjected to violence, and guidance in helping her obtain additional counselling and services;
- informed decision-making.

Clinical skills:

- anatomy and physiology relevant to pregnancy and abortion;
- pre-procedure assessment (e.g. medical history, examinations, pregnancy dating);
- STI screening;
- cervical dilatation;
- uterine evacuation;
- infection prevention;
- pain management;
- recognition and management of complications of abortion;
- management and care following the procedure, including provision of contraceptive information, counselling and methods;
- criteria for referral and referral procedures.

Administrative/managerial issues and quality assurance:

- organization of services to ensure efficient patient flow while maintaining privacy and confidentiality;
- record-keeping and reporting of service statistics;
- practices for maintaining privacy and confidentiality;
- logistics, equipment and inventory management;
- monitoring, evaluation, and quality improvement/assurance;
- mechanisms for effective referral and transport;
- standards for supervision.

3.5.1 Monitoring

Monitoring oversees the processes of implementing services, including changes over time. Routine monitoring can assist managers and supervisors to identify and manage, or avoid, problems before they become serious or overwhelming. Good monitoring includes listening to service providers, who can have important recommendations to improve the quality of care. Well-designed monitoring enables facility managers and staff supervisors to give feedback on problems to staff and to engage staff in a participatory process to implement solutions. At the facility level, mechanisms for monitoring services include analysis of routine service statistics, case reviews, logbook reviews, observation, checklists, facility assessments, maternal death and near-miss audits, and obtaining feedback from service users to improve the quality of care. Routine abortion-service statistics include: the age and number of women provided an induced abortion by method (vacuum aspiration, medical abortion, D&E) and the gestational age of pregnancy.

Monitoring national indicators of safe abortion is important and has been largely neglected (*35*). The introduction of abortion-specific indicators and service statistics should be developed within the context of monitoring the national maternal and reproductive health programme. Health-facility data on abortion services can be integrated into existing management information systems (e.g. forms, logbooks, supply stock records, checklists, patient records, daily activity registers) rather than creating separate ones (*36*, *37*). The WHO indicators for safe abortion care (*38*) are shown in Table 3.2.

3.5.2 Quality assurance and quality improvement

Quality assurance and improvement encompasses planned and systematic processes for identifying measureable outcomes based on national standards and guidelines and the perspectives of health-service users and care providers, collecting data that reflect the extent to which the outcomes are achieved, and providing feedback to programme managers and service providers. Quality-improvement processes should attempt to identify and address both individual and organizational barriers to the achievement of good quality of care (*39–41*). For abortion care, the goal is to promote change for continuous improvement as part of maintaining good-quality services that respond to the needs of health-care providers, as well as the health-care needs and rights of women. Quality improvement involves ongoing monitoring of routine service delivery, provider performance and patient outcomes, as well as periodic assessments conducted at facility level (*42*).

3.5.3 Evaluation

Evaluation is the systematic assessment of service-delivery processes and outcomes. Comprehensive evaluation requires multiple data sources, including service statistics, feedback from health-care providers and from women and communities served, and financial records. Programme evaluators can focus their attention on three key areas related to policies, programmes and services: access; availability; and quality of care. Examples of a range of issues and questions to consider for periodic assessment and evaluation are highlighted in Box 3.3. Answering these questions can provide information that will enable policy-makers and programme managers to better understand and overcome existing barriers to access and improve the quality of care.

Table 3.2. Indicators for safe abortion care[a]

Area	Indicator	Type of measure	Type of indicator (core[b], additional[c])	Source of data
Access: availability	Number of facilities offering safe abortion services per 500 000 population	Rate	Additional	HIS[d]
	Health-care providers trained to provide safe abortion services to the full extent of the law	Percentage	Additional	Survey (facility)
	Population living within 2 hours travel time from a facility providing safe abortion services	Percentage	Additional	Survey (population)
Access: information	Population with correct knowledge of the legal status of abortion	Percentage	Additional	Survey (population)
	Health-care personnel with correct knowledge of the legal status of abortion	Percentage	Additional	Survey (facility)
Access: quality	Service-delivery points that use WHO-recommended methods for induced abortion	Percentage	Additional	Survey (facility)
	Service-delivery points that use WHO-recommended methods for management of abortion complications	Percentage	Additional	Survey (facility)
Outcome/ impact	Obstetric and gynaecological admissions due to abortion	Percentage	Core	HIS
	Hospitalization rate for unsafe abortion per 1000 women	Rate	Additional	HIS
	Abortions per 1000 live births	Ratio	Core	HIS/survey (population)
	Maternal deaths attributed to abortion	Percentage	Core	HIS/survey (special)/vital registration

[a] Other indicators relevant to achieving universal access to reproductive health can be found in reference *38*.

[b] Indicators that all countries should report.

[c] Indicators that countries could report based on their special needs, contextual characteristics, and capabilities (e.g. when coverage for core data is high).

[d] Health information system.

Table adapted from reference *38*.

Questions and issues to consider for periodic assessment and evaluation of abortion services

These questions and issues are for assessment purposes only; for relevant WHO recommendations see Chapters 2, 3 and 4.

Access to safe abortion services

What are the legal grounds for induced abortion?

- on request;
- socioeconomic reasons;
- health (unspecified; as defined by WHO; or with specific conditions);
- mental health (unspecified or with specific conditions);
- physical health (unspecified or with specific conditions);
- rape;
- incest;
- preservation of life.

What are the costs of abortion services to women?

- official fees:
  - provider fees;
  - facility fees;
- informal fees for health-care providers;
- transportation costs;
- accommodation costs;
- opportunity costs;
- private insurance coverage;
- social welfare coverage.

Are permissions from third parties required before performing abortion?

- parental/guardian or spousal/partner authorization;
- authorization of medical commissions;
- authorization by more than one specialist or physician.

Availability of safe abortion services

Are there enough facilities to provide safe care for all women seeking abortion?

- number of facilities offering safe abortion services per 500 000 population.

What are the facility costs of providing safe abortion care?

- provider time;
- equipment/instruments and supplies;
- medications;
- in-service training;
- other capital and recurring costs.

What abortion statistics are available?

- total number of obstetric/gynaecological admissions;
- total number of induced abortions;
- total number of immediate and delayed complications;
- percentage of complications requiring hospitalization;
- total number of presenting complications (as a result of unsafe or spontaneous abortion).

What abortion methods are available and utilized?

For pregnancies of gestational age <12–14 weeks:

- vacuum aspiration;
- mifepristone and misoprostol;
- misoprostol alone;
- dilatation and curettage.

box 3.3 continued

For pregnancies of gestational age >12–14 weeks:

- dilatation and evacuation;
- mifepristone and misoprostol;
- misoprostol alone;
- instillation with hypertonic saline;
- ethacridine lactate.

Quality of care

Do abortion providers have the competencies required to perform safe abortion?

- confirmation of pregnancy;
- estimation of gestational age;
- appropriate surgical procedure technique;
- appropriate pain management;
- appropriate medical abortion regimen;
- appropriate follow-up.

Are good infection-prevention practices routinely followed?

- standard precautions routinely followed;
- no-touch technique employed for surgical methods;
- initial soaking of used instruments;
- instrument cleaning;
- high-level disinfection or sterilization of medical instruments;
- prophylactic antibiotics administered for surgical methods.

What pain-management options are available and what pain management is actually provided?

- verbal relaxation techniques;
- analgesia;
- local anaesthesia;
- sedation;
- general anaesthesia.

What contraceptive methods are available and what methods are provided?

- barrier methods:
  - condoms;
  - cervical barriers;
- fertility-based awareness methods;
- hormonal methods:
  - pills;
  - vaginal ring;
  - skin patch;
  - injectables;
  - implants;
- IUDs;
- sterilization;
- emergency contraceptives.

What information, education and communication material is available and what information is routinely provided?

- for the procedure;
- for follow-up care;
- for contraception;
- for other needs.

Is counselling routinely offered?

- for the procedure;
- for follow-up care;
- for contraception;
- for other needs.

Are services managed effectively and efficiently?

- in-service training routinely provided;
- adequate supervision;
- sufficient financing;
- sufficient procurement, distribution and restocking of instruments, medications and supplies;
- adequate management information systems;
- mechanisms for quality improvement/assurance;
- mechanisms for monitoring and evaluation of services.

box 3.3 continued

Is an adequate referral system in place for:

- induced abortion (especially for cases of conscientious objection to service provision);
- management of complications;
- contraception;
- reproductive tract infections;
- gender-based violence.

Are all aspects of a woman's privacy maintained regarding her abortion?

- visual privacy during examination and procedure;
- auditory privacy during counselling, examination and procedure;
- non-essential staff excluded from the room during the procedure;
- offer of home use of misoprostol following provision of mifepristone;
- adequate toilets with privacy;
- discreet signage for location of abortion services.

Is a woman's confidentiality protected regarding her abortion?

- access to medical records restricted;
- confidentiality maintained for all women, including adolescents.

Are delays for seeking care minimized?

- no mandatory waiting periods;
- time required between requesting and scheduling the procedure;
- time waiting for the procedure;
- total time in hospital/clinic.

Do other potential service-delivery barriers exist?

- requirements for HIV and other tests that are not clinically indicated;
- mandatory counselling beyond provision of adequate information relevant to the woman's abortion care;
- requirement for mandatory ultrasound prior to abortion;
- requirement for women to listen to fetal heartbeat prior to abortion;
- requirement for listing induced abortion on permanent medical records, where confidentiality cannot be assured.

Women's perspectives about abortion services

- were the abortion provider and clinic staff friendly and professional?
- was sufficient information provided about the procedure, contraception and follow-up?
- did the woman have an opportunity to ask questions?
- were questions appropriately answered?
- was privacy protected?
- would the woman recommend the facility?
- would the woman recommend the provider?

Provider perspectives

- does the organization and implementation of abortion services meet evidence-based standards?
- is the quality of care sufficient?
- how could job satisfaction be improved?
- is supervisor support adequate?
- are work incentives (e.g. salary, fees, professional development opportunities) sufficient?

3.6 Financing

Health-service budgets should include sufficient funds for the following types of costs:

- equipment, medications and supplies required to provide safe abortion care;
- staff time;
- training programmes and supervision;
- infrastructure upgrades;
- record-keeping;
- monitoring and evaluation.

To the extent that the abortion programme can be integrated within the national maternal and reproductive health programme, the marginal costs of putting in place or improving abortion services will be minimized. In general, safe abortion services require few, if any, additional provider skills, medications, equipment or supplies from those that should already be available for emergency obstetric and gynaecological care.

3.6.1 Cost to the facility or health system

The provision of safe, legal abortion is considerably less costly than treating the complications of unsafe abortion (43–47). Costs for providing abortion care with vacuum aspiration include infrequent, modest capital investments, such as a suction machine or MVA equipment; an examination table; a steam sterilizer or autoclave; renovation of waiting, consultation and recovery rooms; and toilets. Recurrent costs include those associated with purchasing instruments and supplies that will need to be restocked regularly, such as cannulae and manual vacuum aspirators; antiseptic solutions and high-level disinfectants used for instrument processing; and drugs for pain management, infection prevention and medical abortion.

Decisions made about which abortion methods to offer and how to organize services directly influence the cost of providing services and their affordability. Two organizational issues are of particular importance: preferential use of vacuum aspiration or medical abortion over D&C, and informing women to come earlier rather than later for induced abortion.

- Switching from D&C to vacuum aspiration or medical abortion for uterine evacuation is safer for the woman and can reduce health-system costs (23, 24). Vacuum aspiration can be performed by a trained midlevel health-care provider in an office or examination room, whereas D&C is often performed in an operating theatre by a physician. Also, vacuum aspiration usually requires less medication for pain than D&C (23, 47, 48).

- If the health system effectively informs women to come early in pregnancy for abortion, the use of lower-cost early procedures increases and use of costlier later procedures declines. For example, the introduction of combination mifepristone and misoprostol has been associated with population shifts to abortion at earlier gestational ages (49, 50). Home use of misoprostol contributes to greater flexibility for the woman and decreased staff and facility utilization. This also enables services to be provided at lower levels of the health system and thus closer to women's residences, thereby decreasing travel and time-associated costs.

3.6.2 Making services affordable for women

In many settings, national health insurance schemes do not exist or do not cover large portions of the population or do not include abortion within the benefit package. Other sources of financing of health services are often employed, including requiring contributions from individuals who use the health system. WHO recommends that payments from individuals for health services be collected as a type of prepayment, rather than at the time of service delivery (51). However, in many settings, user fees are customarily charged and can be an important barrier to services for poor women and adolescents. In addition, women seeking abortion may be expected to pay substantial informal fees (charges made by providers on top of the official health-system charges) which, when combined with travel expenses and opportunity costs such as time lost from paid employment, pose a barrier for many women. The barrier of high costs to women is likely to generate higher costs for the health system, by increasing the number of women who attempt to self-induce abortion or go to unsafe providers and, as a result, require hospitalization for serious complications (52, 53).

The respect, protection, and fulfilment of human rights require that women can access legal abortion services regardless of their ability to pay. Financing mechanisms should ensure equitable access to good-quality services (54). Where user fees are charged for abortion, such fees should be matched to women's ability to pay, and procedures should be developed for exempting the poor and adolescents from paying for services. As far as possible, abortion services should be mandated for coverage under insurance plans. Abortion should never be denied or delayed because of a woman's inability to pay. Furthermore, all facilities should have procedures in place to ensure that informal charges are not imposed by staff.

3.7 The process of planning and managing safe abortion care

Establishing abortion services or strengthening access to and the quality of care of existing abortion services at national or subnational level, to the full extent of the law, should be driven by dedicated and committed stakeholders who can provide strong leadership, identify and recruit other stakeholders, and mobilize funding and technical assistance to support a wide range of activities. Ideally, leadership would be situated in the ministry/department of health or another institution with the mandate to influence and mobilize national action. Important stakeholders include: representatives from other government ministries or departments, such as education, gender and women's affairs, justice, local government, social welfare, and youth affairs; medical universities; professional health associations – particularly those of obstetrician-gynaecologists but also those of family physicians, nurses, midwives and pharmacists; other public health cadres; women's health advocates; nongovernmental organizations focused on women, youth, health, and human rights; other relevant representatives of civil society; and key development partners (55).

Principles underlying the process of improving access to and the quality of abortion care include the following. The process should be: country owned and country led; evidence based; inclusive of multiple perspectives; participatory; embracing sex and gender equality and non-discrimination; health and human-rights based; and system focused (55).

Strengthening abortion services is a political and managerial challenge, in addition to being a clinical or technical task. One methodology that has been used effectively is the *WHO Strategic Approach to strengthening sexual and reproductive health policies and programmes (55–60)*. The Strategic Approach begins with the creation of an assessment team representing a broad range of stakeholders, such as those mentioned above, who conduct a field-based assessment to identify and prioritize needs related

Planning and managing safe abortion care

to abortion and contraceptive-service access, availability and quality of care. Based on the findings and recommendations of the assessment team, a package of policy and programme interventions are implemented on a limited scale to provide local evidence of feasibility, effectiveness and acceptability. If successful, the interventions are then scaled-up to have broader impact.

Whatever methods are used, it is important that actions to strengthen policies and services are based on a thorough understanding of the service-delivery system, the needs of providers, the needs of women, and the existing social, cultural, legal, political and economic context. It is also important that multiple perspectives are incorporated. This helps to ensure that recommendations and plans based on the assessment will be broadly acceptable and therefore more likely to be implemented. It is particularly important to include the perspectives on services from users and potential users, as they are the main source of identifying barriers to service use. It is also important that the assessment examines people's access to sexual and reproductive health services generally, and specifically their access to contraceptive information, counselling and methods, since these are important determinants of the incidence of unintended pregnancy.

3.7.1 Assessing the current situation

Local contexts in need of improved abortion care vary considerably in terms of scale – from system level to individual facilities – and with regard to specific areas requiring strengthening. For improving abortion care at facility level, see Section 3.5.2. At the national or health-system level, the first step in assessing the current situation related to unintended pregnancy and abortion involves collecting and analysing existing information on:

- laws on sexuality, contraception, and abortion;
- ratified human rights agreements;
- access to and availability of contraceptives;
- sexuality education;
- service-delivery standards and guidelines;
- curricula of health-care and other relevant professional schools;
- availability of abortion-related medical devices and drugs;
- facility- and national-level health statistics;
- demographic/reproductive health surveys;
- relevant research studies;
- health insurance or other measures to reduce out-of-pocket expenditures for abortion services.

Following a thorough compilation and review of existing information, the field team can develop discussion guides for use with policy-makers, health-care providers, women and other relevant community members. Guiding questions for a field assessment might include how policies, programmes and services can be strengthened to:

- prevent unintended pregnancy;
- improve access to and the availability of safe abortion;
- improve the quality of abortion care.

Exploring each of these in detail will help the team to identify and prioritize the most critical policy and programmatic needs. A field guide is available with more detailed information about the process of conducting a strategic assessment (61) (available from: http://www.who.int/reproductivehealth/publications/familyplanning/RHR_02_11).

3.7.2 Introducing interventions to strengthen abortion care

New policy and programme interventions should be guided by evidence-based best practices. Much of the evidence for abortion policies and programmes is reflected in the recommendations presented in this guidance document. However, programme managers often want to be assured through local evidence of the feasibility, effectiveness, acceptability and cost of the introduction of changes in policy and programme design, or service-delivery practices, prior to committing resources for their implementation on a larger scale. Even when interventions are based on accepted international best practices, some evidence of the capacity for local implementation and acceptability among community members is likely to be necessary to facilitate scaling-up. Depending on the quality of evidence required by policy-makers, testing of the intervention(s) could range from simple pilot or demonstration projects to more rigorous implementation research incorporating quasi-experimental designs.

3.7.3 Scaling-up policy and programmatic interventions

Scaling-up involves expanding the health system's capacity for implementation of policy and programme interventions that have been demonstrated to improve access to and the quality of abortion care, in order to achieve population-level impact. Too often, scaling-up is considered a matter of routine programme implementation that does not need special attention. Once a package of interventions has proved to be successful in a pilot or demonstration project, it is expected to be taken up by a health system and spread throughout, based on the assumption that success in the pilot phase is sufficient to catalyse large-scale change. While this

sometimes happens, more frequently it does not. Successful scaling-up requires systematic planning, management, guidance and support for the process by which interventions are expanded and institutionalized. Scaling-up also requires sufficient human and financial resources to support the process. Guidance for the development of comprehensive strategies for scaling-up and for management of the process is available from WHO and ExpandNet (*62–64*; http://www.expandnet.net/tools).

Systematic approaches to scaling-up recognize that the process takes place in a context of "real-world" complexity, with multiple and often competing players and interests. Attention to technical concerns is essential, but equally important are the political, managerial and ownership issues that come into play, since interventions to improve access and quality of care often call for changes in values as well as practices. This is especially relevant for an issue such as safe abortion.

Health systems are often limited in their ability to deliver the range of needed services that current policies mandate, and integrating a new set of interventions can place additional burdens on an already stressed system. Yet, when scaling-up is approached systematically and with sufficient financial and human resources to support it, the process can be successful and contribute to achieving the goal of universal access to reproductive health care, including safe abortion.

References

1. *Women and health: today's evidence, tomorrow's agenda*. Geneva, World Health Organization, 2009.

2. Myers JE, Seif MW. Global perspective of legal abortion – trends, analysis and accessibility. *Best Practice and Research Clinical Obstetrics and Gynaecology*, 2010, 24:457–466.

3. Warriner IK et al. Can midlevel health-care providers administer early medical abortion as safely and effectively as doctors? A randomised controlled equivalence trial in Nepal. *Lancet*, 2011, 377:1155–1161.

4. Kishen M, Stedman Y. The role of advanced nurse practitioners in the availability of abortion services. *Best Practice and Research Clinical Obstetrics and Gynaecology*, 2010, 24:569–578.

5. Jejeebhoy S et al. Can nurses perform MVA as safely and effectively as physicians? Evidence from India. *Contraception*, 2011, 84:615–621.

6. Warriner IK et al. Rates of complication in first-trimester manual vacuum abortion done by doctors and mid-level providers in South Africa and Vietnam: a randomised controlled equivalence trial. *Lancet*, 2006, 368(9551):1965–1972.

7. Shearer JC, Walker DG, Vlassoff M. Cost of post-abortion care in low- and middle-income countries. *International Journal of Gynecology and Obstetrics*, 2009, 108:165–169.

8. Bracken H. Family Planning Association of India (FPAI)/Gynuity Health Projects Research Group for Simplifying Medical Abortion in India. Home administration of misoprostol for early medical abortion in India. *International Journal of Gynaecology and Obstetrics*, 2010, 108:228–232.

9. Shannon C et al. Regimens of misoprostol with mifepristone for early medical abortion: a randomised trial. *British Journal of Obstetrics and Gynaecology*, 2006, 113:621–628.

10. Ngo TD et al. *Comparative effectiveness, safety and acceptability of medical abortion at home and in a clinic: a systematic review*. Geneva, World Health Organization, 2011 (Report no. 89).

11. *Complications of abortion: technical and managerial guidelines for prevention and treatment*. Geneva, World Health Organization, 1995.

12. *Sexual and reproductive health care core competencies for primary health*. Geneva, World Health Organization, 2011.

13. Freedman M et al. Comparison of complication rates in first trimester abortions performed by physician assistants and physicians. *American Journal of Public Health*, 1986, 76:550–554.

14. Greenslade F et al. Summary of clinical and programmatic experience with manual vacuum aspiration. *IPAS Advances in Abortion Care*, 1993, 3(2):1–4.

15. Berer M. Provision of abortion by mid-level providers: international policy, practice and perspectives. *Bulletin of the World Health Organization*, 2009, 87:58–63.

16. Iyengar SD. Introducing medical abortion within the primary health system: comparison with other health interventions and commodities. *Reproductive Health Matters*, 2005, 13:13–19.

17. Yarnell J, Swica Y, Winikoff B. Non-physician clinicians can safely provide first trimester medical abortion. *Reproductive Health Matters*, 2009, 17:61–69.

18. Cook RJ, Dickens BM. Human rights dynamics of abortion law reform. *Human Rights Quarterly*, 2003, 25:1–59.

19. *General Comment No. 4: Adolescent health and development in the context of the Convention on the Rights of the Child*. Geneva, Committee on the Rights of the Child, 2003 (Report no. CRC/GC/2003/4).

20. World Health Organization and The Office of the United Nations High Commissioner for Refugees. *Clinical management of survivors of rape. A guide to the development of protocols for use in refugee and internally displaced person situations*. Geneva, World Health Organization, 2002.

21. Cook RJ, Erdman JN, Dickens BM. Respecting adolescents' confidentiality and reproductive and sexual choices. *International Journal of Gynecology and Obstetrics*, 2007, 92:182–187.

22. Billings D et al. Constructing access to legal abortion services in Mexico City. *Reproductive Health Matters*, 2002, 10:87–95.

23. Johnson BR et al. Costs and resource utilization for the treatment of incomplete abortion in Kenya and Mexico. *Social Science and Medicine*, 1993, 36:1443–1453.

24. Jowett M. Safe motherhood interventions in low-income countries: an economic justification and evidence of cost effectiveness. *Health Policy*, 2000, 53:201–228.

25. *WHO model list of essential medicines*, 16th ed. Geneva, World Health Organization, 2010.

26. *Model certificate of a pharmaceutical product*. Geneva, World Health Organization, 2011 (http://www.who.int/medicines/areas/quality_safety/regulation_legislation/certification/modelcertificate/en/index.html, accessed 1 September 2011).

27. Mitchell EMH et al. Building alliances from ambivalence: evaluation of abortion values clarification workshops with stakeholders in South Africa. *African Journal of Reproductive Health*, 2005, 9:89–99.

28. *The abortion option: a values clarification guide for health care professionals*. Washington, DC, National Abortion Federation, 2005.

29. Turner KL, Chapman Page K. *Abortion attitude transformation: a values clarification toolkit for global audiences*. Chapel Hill, Ipas, 2008.

30. Billings D et al. Midwives and comprehensive postabortion care in Ghana. In: Huntington D, Piet-Pelon NJ, eds. *Postabortion care: lessons from operations research*. New York, Population Council, 1999:141–158.

31. Dickson-Tetteh K et al. Abortion care services provided by registered midwives in South Africa: a report on the midwifery training program. *International Family Planning Perspectives*, 2002, 28:144–150.

32. *Senegal: postabortion care. Train more providers in postabortion care*. New York, Population Council, 2000.

33. *PRIME postabortion care. Program for International Training in Health (INTRAH)*. Chapel Hill, University of North Carolina, 2001.

34. Yumkella F, Githiori F. *Expanding opportunities for postabortion care at the community level through private nurse-midwives in Kenya*. Chapel Hill, Program for International Training in Health (INTRAH), 2000.

35. Healy J, Otsea K, Benson J. Counting abortions so that abortion counts: indicators for monitoring the availability and use of abortion care services. *International Journal of Gynaecology and Obstetrics*, 2006, 95:209–220.

36. *Packages of interventions for family planning, safe abortion care, maternal, newborn and child health*. Geneva, World Health Organization, 2010.

37. *Monitoring emergency obstetric care: a handbook*. Geneva, World Health Organization, 2009.

38. World Health Organization, UNFPA. *National-level monitoring of the achievement of universal access to reproductive health: conceptual and practical considerations and related indicators*. Geneva, World Health Organization, 2008.

39. Mulligan EA. Striving for excellence in abortion services. *Australian Health Review*, 2006, 30:468–473.

40. Foy R et al. Theory-based identification of barriers to quality improvement: induced abortion care. *Journal for Quality in Health Care*, 2005, 17:147–155.

41. Morrison J. Audit of the care of women requesting induced abortion. *Journal of Obstetrics and Gynaecology*, 2003, 23:521–524.

42. EngenderHealth, Ipas. *COPE® for comprehensive abortion care: a toolbook to accompany the COPE handbook*. EngenderHealth Quality Improvement Series. New York, EngenderHealth, 2009.

43. Billings DL, Benson J. Postabortion care in Latin America: policy and service recommendations from a decade of operations research. *Health Policy and Planning*, 2005, 20:158–166.

44. Johnston HB, Gallo MF, Benson J. Reducing the costs to health systems of unsafe abortion: a comparison of four strategies. *Journal of Family Planning and Reproductive Health Care*, 2007, 33:250–257.

45. Vlassoff M et al. *Economic impact of unsafe abortion-related morbidity and mortality: evidence and estimation challenges*. Brighton, Institute of Development Studies, 2008 (Report no. 59).

Planning and managing safe abortion care

46. Levin C et al. Exploring the costs and economic consequences of unsafe abortion in Mexico City before legalisation. *Reproductive Health Matters*, 2009, 17:120–132.

47. Hu D et al. Cost-effectiveness analysis of unsafe abortion. *African Journal of Reproductive Health*, 2010, 14:85–103.

48. Grimes D et al. Abortion in the seventies. In: *The Joint Program for the Study of Abortion/CDC – a preliminary report.* Washington, DC, National Abortion Federation, 1977:41–46.

49. Jones R, Henshaw R. Mifepristone for early medical abortion: experiences in France, Great Britain and Sweden. *Perspectives in Sexual and Reproductive Health*, 2002, 34:154–161.

50. Finer L, Wei J. Effect of mifepristone on abortion access in the United States. *Obstetrics and Gynecology*, 2009, 114:623–630.

51. *Performance incentives for health care providers.* Geneva, World Health Organization, 2010 (Discussion Paper 1).

52. Duggal R. The political economy of abortion in India: cost and expenditure patterns. *Reproductive Health Matters*, 2004, 12(24 Suppl.):130–137.

53. Naghma-e-Rehan. Cost of the treatment of complications of unsafe abortion in public hospitals. *Journal of the Pakistan Medical Association*, 2011, 61:169–172.

54. Resolution WHA58.33. Sustainable health financing, universal coverage and social health insurance. In: *Fifty-eighth World Health Assembly, 16–25 May 2005. Geneva*, World Health Organization, 2005 (WHA58/2005/REC/1).

55. *The WHO Strategic Approach to strengthening sexual and reproductive health policies and programmes.* Geneva, World Health Organization, 2007.

56. *Abortion in Viet Nam: an assessment of policy, programme and research issues.* Geneva, World Health Organization, 1999.

57. Johnson BR, Horga M, Fajans P. A strategic assessment of abortion and contraception in Romania. *Reproductive Health Matters*, 2004, 12(24 Suppl.):184–194.

58. Tsogt B, Kisghgee S, Johnson BR. Applying the WHO Strategic Approach to strengthening first and second trimester abortion services in Mongolia. *Reproductive Health Matters*, 2008, 16(31 Suppl.):127–134.

59. *Strategic assessment of policy, quality and access to contraception and abortion in the Republic of Macedonia.* Skopje, Republic Institute for Health Protection, 2008.

60. Jackson E et al. A strategic assessment of unsafe abortion in Malawi. *Reproductive Health Matters*, 2011, 19:133–143.

61. *Making decisions about contraceptive introduction. A guide for conducting assessments to broaden contraceptive choice and improve quality of care.* Geneva, World Health Organization, 2002.

62. World Health Organization, ExpandNet. *Practical guidance for scaling up health service innovations.* Geneva, World Health Organization, 2009.

63. World Health Organization, ExpandNet. *Nine steps for developing a scaling-up strategy.* Geneva, World Health Organization, 2010.

64. World Health Organization, ExpandNet. *Beginning with the end in mind: planning pilot projects and programmatic resesarch for scaling up success.* Geneva, World Health Organization, 2011.

Chapter 4

CHAPTER 4
Legal and policy considerations

Summary

- Unsafe abortion is one of the four main causes of maternal mortality and morbidity. One of the reasons for unsafe abortion is because safe abortion services are frequently not available, even when they are legal for a variety of indications in almost all countries.

- International, regional and national human rights bodies and courts increasingly recommend decriminalization of abortion, and provision of abortion care, to protect a woman's life and health, and in cases of rape, based on a woman's complaint. Ensuring that laws, even when restrictive, are interpreted and implemented to promote and protect women's health is essential.

- Additional barriers, that may or may not be codified in law, often impede women from reaching the services for which they are eligible and contribute to unsafe abortion. These barriers include lack of access to information; requiring third-party authorization; restricting the type of health-care providers and facilities that can lawfully provide services; failing to guarantee access to affordable services; failing to guarantee confidentiality and privacy; and allowing conscientious objection without referrals on the part of health-care providers and facilities.

- An enabling regulatory and policy environment is needed to ensure that every woman who is legally eligible has ready access to good-quality abortion services. Policies should be geared to respecting, protecting and fulfilling the human rights of women, to achieving positive health outcomes for women, to providing good-quality contraceptive and family planning information and services, and to meeting the particular needs of poor women, adolescents, rape survivors and women living with HIV.

4.1 Women's health and human rights

Unsafe abortion accounts for 13% of maternal deaths (1), and 20% of the total mortality and disability burden due to pregnancy and childbirth (2). Almost all deaths and morbidity from unsafe abortion occur in countries where abortion is severely restricted in law and in practice. Every year, about 47 000 women die from complications of unsafe abortion (3), an estimated 5 million women suffer temporary or permanent disability, including infertility (4). Where there are few restrictions on access to safe abortion, deaths and illness are dramatically reduced (5). This chapter highlights the inextricable link between women's health and human rights and the need for laws and policies that promote and protect both.

Most governments have ratified legally binding international treaties and conventions that protect human rights, including the right to the highest attainable standard of health, the right to non-discrimination, the right to life, the right to liberty and the right to security of the person, the right to be free from inhuman and degrading treatment, and the right to education and information. These rights are further recognized and defined in regional treaties, enacted in national constitutions and laws of many countries.

In consideration of these human rights, governments agreed in the United Nations International Conference on Population and Development, 1999 (ICPD+5) review and appraisal process that "in circumstances where abortion is not against the law, health systems should train and equip health-service providers and should take other measures to ensure that such abortion is safe and accessible. Additional measures should be taken to safeguard women's health" (6). The original document, *Safe abortion: technical and policy guidance for health systems*, published by the World Health Organization (WHO) in 2003 started from this mandate (7).

Over the past 15 years, human rights have been increasingly applied by international and regional human rights bodies and national courts, including

---

BOX 4.1

Examples of application of human rights to safe abortion, in the context of comprehensive reproductive health care, by international and regional human rights bodies

Human rights, as they are enshrined in international and regional treaties and in national constitutions, and the output of United Nations treaty monitoring bodies, including their general comments/recommendations and concluding observations to States, as well as regional and national court decisions form a reference system for human rights accountability at international, regional and national levels. They give clear guidance to States (in the case of concluding observations, to individual States) on the measures to be taken to ensure the respect, protection and fulfilment of human rights.

UN treaty monitoring bodies, regional and national courts have given increasing attention to the issue of abortion during the past decades, including maternal mortality due to unsafe abortion, criminalization of abortion, and restrictive legislation that leads women to obtain illegal and unsafe abortions. Increasingly they have called upon States to provide comprehensive sexual and reproductive health information and services to women and adolescents, eliminate regulatory and administrative barriers that impede women's access to safe abortion services and provide treatment for abortion complications. If they do not do so, States may not meet their treaty and constitutional obligations to respect, protect and fulfil the right to life, the right to non-discrimination, the right to the highest attainable standard of health, the right to be free from cruel, inhuman and degrading treatment and the rights to privacy, confidentiality, information and education. UN treaty monitoring body recommendations and regional court decisions to States include the following examples: [1]

Ensuring comprehensive legal grounds for abortion

- Take action to prevent unsafe abortion, including by amending restrictive laws that threaten women's, including adolescents', lives (9).
- Provide legal abortion in cases where the continued pregnancy endangers the health of women, including adolescents (10).
- Provide legal abortion in cases of rape and incest (11).
- Amend laws that criminalize medical procedures, including abortion, needed only by women and/or that punish women who undergo those procedures (12).

---

[1] The detailed references reflect a growing number of UN treaty monitoring body general comments/recommendations and concluding observations, as well as regional treaty provisions and regional court decisions related to abortion.

the United Nations treaty monitoring bodies in the context of abortion (see Box 4.1). They recommended that States reform laws that criminalize medical procedures that are needed only by women, and that punish women who undergo these procedures (8), both of which are applicable in the case of abortion. In order to protect women's health and human rights these human rights bodies recommended that States should make all efforts to ensure that women do not have to undergo life-threatening clandestine abortions and that abortion should be legal at a minimum when continuation of the pregnancy endangers the life (9) and health (10) of the woman and in cases of rape and incest (11). They also recommended that States should ensure timely and affordable access to good-quality health services, which should be delivered in a way that ensures that a woman gives her fully informed consent, respects her dignity, guarantees her confidentiality, and is sensitive to her needs and perspectives (8).

---

box 4.1 continued

Planning and managing safe abortion care

- Ensure timely access to a range of good-quality sexual and reproductive health services, including for adolescents, which are delivered in a way that ensures a woman's fully informed consent, respects her dignity, guarantees her confidentiality and is sensitive to her needs and perspectives (13).
- Reduce maternal morbidity and mortality in adolescents, particularly caused by early pregnancy and unsafe abortion practices, and develop and implement programmes that provide access to sexual and reproductive health services, including family planning, contraception and safe abortion services where abortion is not against the law (14).
- Provide information on sexual and reproductive health, and mechanisms to ensure that all women, including adolescents, have access to information about legal abortion services (15).

Eliminating regulatory, policy and access barriers

- Remove third-party authorization requirements that interfere with women's and adolescents' right to make decisions about reproduction and to exercise control over their bodies (16).
- Eliminate barriers that impede women's access to health services, such as high fees for health-care services, the requirement for preliminary authorization by spouse, parent or hospital authorities, long distances from health facilities and the absence of convenient and affordable public transport, and also ensure that the exercise of conscientious objection does not prevent individuals from accessing services to which they are legally entitled (17).
- Implement a legal and/or policy framework that enables women to access abortion where the medical procedure is permitted under the law (18).

Providing treatment of abortion complications

- Provide timely treatment for abortion complications regardless of the law on induced abortion, to protect a woman's life and health (19).
- Eliminate the practice of extracting confessions for prosecution purposes from women seeking emergency medical care as a result of illegal abortion and the legal requirement for doctors and other health-care personnel to report cases of women who have undergone abortion (20).

Given the clear link between access to safe abortion and women's health, it is recommended that laws and policies should respect and protect women's health and their human rights.

4.2 Laws and their implementation within the context of human rights

Legal restrictions on abortion do not result in fewer abortions nor do they result in significant increases in birth rates (21, 22). Conversely, laws and policies that facilitate access to safe abortion do not increase the rate or number of abortions. The principle effect is to shift previously clandestine, unsafe procedures to legal and safe ones (21, 23).

Restricting legal access to abortion does not decrease the need for abortion, but it is likely to increase the number of women seeking illegal and unsafe abortions, leading to increased morbidity and mortality. Legal restrictions also lead many women to seek services in other countries/states (24, 25), which is costly, delays access and creates social inequities. Restricting abortion, with the intent of boosting population has been well documented in several countries. In each case, abortion restrictions resulted in an increase of illegal and unsafe abortions and pregnancy-related mortality, with insignificant net increase in the population (26–29).

Abortion laws began to be liberalized, through legislation and/or through broader legal interpretations and applications, in the first part of the 20th century when the extent of the public health problem of unsafe abortion began to be recognized. Dating from the late 1960s, there has been a trend towards liberalization of the legal grounds for abortion (30). Since 1985, over 36 countries have liberalized their abortion laws, while only a few countries have imposed further restrictions in their laws (31). These reforms have come about through both judicial and legislative action.

Evidence increasingly shows that, where abortion is legal on broad socioeconomic grounds and on a woman's request, and where safe services are accessible, both unsafe abortion and abortion-related mortality and morbidity are reduced (32–35) (see Figure 4.1).

Fifty-seven countries, representing almost 40% of the world's women, allow abortion upon request of the pregnant woman (31, 36). In this context, the ultimate decision on whether to continue or terminate her pregnancy belongs to the woman alone. In some criminal or penal codes abortion throughout pregnancy, or up to a set gestational limit, is no longer subject to criminal regulation, and has been removed as a distinct offence. In these situations, abortion services have usually been integrated into the health system and are governed by the laws, regulations and medical standards that apply to all health services. Approximately 20% of the world's women live in countries that have laws that allow abortion based on a woman's social and economic circumstances (31), including the effect of continued pregnancy on her existing children and other family members.

Nonetheless, across the world, 40% of women of childbearing age live in countries that have highly restrictive laws (31, 37), and/or where abortion, even when lawful, is neither available nor accessible.

Figure 4.1 Deaths attributable to unsafe abortion per 100 000 live births, by legal grounds for abortion

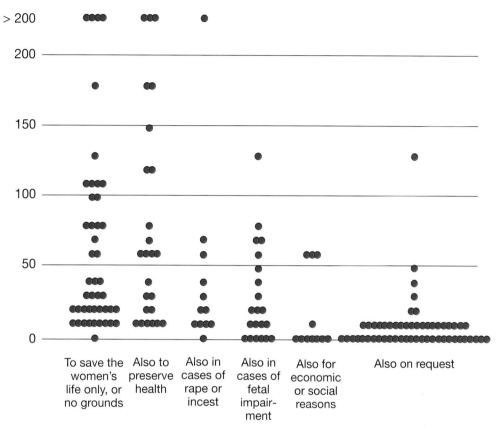

• Every dot represents one country

Reproduced from: *The World Health Report 2008 – primary health care now more than ever.* Geneva, World Health Organization, 2008.

4.2.1 Understanding legal grounds for abortion

4.2.1.1 When there is a threat to the woman's life

Almost all countries allow abortion to be performed to save the life of the pregnant woman. This is consistent with the human right to life, which requires protection by law, including when pregnancy is life-threatening or a pregnant woman's life is otherwise endangered (*9*).

Both medical and social conditions can constitute life-threatening conditions. Some countries provide detailed lists of what they consider life-threatening *medical* conditions. Such lists may be interpreted restrictively or be considered exhaustive, when in fact they are meant to provide illustrations of situations that are considered life-threatening and do not preclude clinical judgement of what is life-threatening for a particular woman. In some cases, physicians argue that it is necessary to provide a safe abortion because, if they did not, the woman would risk her life by going to an unqualified practitioner (*38*). An example of a life-threatening *social* condition is a pregnancy that implicates so-called family "honour". For example, in some societies pregnancy out of wedlock may result in a woman being subjected to physical violence or even killed.

- Even where protecting a woman's life is the only allowable reason for abortion, it is essential that there are trained providers of abortion services, that services are available and known, and that treatment for complications of unsafe abortion is widely available. Saving a woman's life might be necessary at any point in the pregnancy and, when required, abortion should be undertaken as promptly as possible to minimize risks to a woman's health. Treatment of complications from unsafe abortion should be provided in ways that preserve women's dignity and equality.

4.2.1.2 When there is a threat to a woman's health

The fulfilment of human rights requires that women can access safe abortion when it is indicated to protect their health (*10*). Physical health is widely understood to include conditions that aggravate pregnancy and those aggravated by pregnancy. The scope of mental health includes psychological distress or mental suffering caused by, for example, coerced or forced sexual acts and diagnosis of severe fetal impairment (*39*). A woman's social circumstances are also taken into account to assess health risk.

- In many countries, the law does not specify the aspects of health that are concerned but merely states that abortion is permitted to avert risk of injury to the pregnant woman's health. Since all countries that are members of WHO accept its constitutional description of health as "a state of complete physical, mental and social well-being and not merely the absence of disease or infirmity" (*40*), this description of complete health is implied in the interpretation of laws that allow abortion to protect women's health.

4.2.1.3 When pregnancy is the result of rape or incest

The protection of women from cruel, inhuman and degrading treatment requires that those who have become pregnant as the result of coerced or forced sexual acts can lawfully access safe abortion services (*41*). Nearly 50% of countries reflect this standard and permit abortion in the specific case of rape, or more generally where pregnancy is the result of a criminal act, such as in cases of incest (*36*). Some countries require as evidence the woman's report of the act to legal authorities. Others require forensic evidence of sexual penetration or a police investigation to confirm that intercourse was involuntary or exploitative. Delays owing to such requirements can result in women being denied services because they have exceeded gestational age limits prescribed by law. In many contexts, women who have been victims of rape may fear being stigmatized further by the police and others and will therefore avoid reporting the rape at all, thus precluding access to legal abortion. Either situation can lead women to resort to clandestine, unsafe services to terminate their pregnancy.

- Prompt, safe abortion services should be provided on the basis of a woman's complaint rather than requiring forensic evidence or police examination (42, 43). Administrative requirements should be minimized and clear protocols established for both police and health-care providers as this will facilitate referral and access to care (44, 45).

4.2.1.4 When there is fetal impairment

Countries with otherwise restrictive abortion laws are increasingly permitting abortion upon diagnosis of fetal impairment or anomalies due to genetic or other causes. Several countries specify the kinds of impairment, such as those considered to be incompatible with life or independent life, while others provide lists of impairments (36). Such lists tend to be restrictive and are therefore a barrier to women accessing safe abortion services. In some countries, no reference is made in the law to fetal impairment; rather, health protection or social reasons are interpreted to include distress of the pregnant woman caused by the diagnosis of fetal impairment (46, 47).

- Prenatal tests and other medical diagnostic services cannot legally be refused because the woman may decide to terminate her pregnancy. A woman is entitled to know the status of her pregnancy and to act on this information.

4.2.1.5 For economic and social reasons

In countries that permit abortion for economic and social reasons, the legal grounds are interpreted by reference to whether continued pregnancy would affect the actual or foreseeable circumstances of the woman, including her achievement of the highest attainable standard of health. Some laws specify allowable reasons, such as pregnancy outside of marriage, failed contraception, or intellectual disability affecting capacity to care for a child, while others only imply them (48). Laws may also require distress as a result of changed circumstance, for example, the distress of caring and providing for a child additional to existing family members.

4.2.1.6 On request

Nearly a third of UN Member States allow abortion upon the free and informed request of the pregnant woman (36). Allowing abortion on request has emerged as countries have recognized that women seek abortions on one, and often more than one of the above grounds, and they accept all of these as legitimate, without requiring a specific reason. This legal ground recognizes the conditions for a woman's free choice. Most countries that allow abortion on request set limitations for this ground based on duration of pregnancy.

4.2.1.7 Limits on length of pregnancy

Laws or policies that impose time limits on the length of pregnancy for which abortion can be performed may have negative consequences for women who have exceeded the limit. Such policies/laws force some women to seek services from unsafe providers, or self-induce with misoprostol or a less-safe method, or force them to seek services in other countries, which is costly, delays access (thus increasing health risk) and creates social inequities.

In addition, some service-delivery contexts restrict the services they offer by gestational limits that are not evidence based. For example, some countries offer outpatient abortion services only up to 8 weeks gestation when they could be safely provided even after 12–14 weeks gestation (see Chapters 2 and 3). Also some countries offer vacuum aspiration only up to 6 or 8 weeks, when it can be safely provided to 12–14 weeks gestation by trained health-care personnel. These policies also encourage the continued use of less-safe procedures, such as dilatation and curettage.

4.2.2 Legal, regulatory or administrative barriers to safe abortion access in the context of human rights

The legal grounds, and the scope of their interpretation, are only one dimension of the legal and policy environment that affects women's access to safe abortion. Health system and service-delivery barriers as they are explained in Chapter 3 may also be codified in laws, regulations, policies and practices. Laws, policies and practices that restrict access to abortion information and services can deter women from care seeking and create a "chilling effect" (suppression of actions because of fear of reprisals or penalties) for the provision of safe, legal services. Examples of barriers include:

- prohibiting access to information on legal abortion services, or failing to provide public information on the legal status of abortion;

- requiring third-party authorization from one or more medical professionals or a hospital committee, court or police, parent or guardian or a woman's partner or spouse;

- restricting available methods of abortion, including surgical and medical methods through, for instance, lack of regulatory approval for essential medicines;

- restricting the range of health-care providers and facilities that can safely provide services, e.g. to physicians in inpatient facilities with sophisticated equipment;

- failing to assure referral in case of conscientious objection;

- requiring mandatory waiting periods;

- censoring, withholding or intentionally misrepresenting health-related information;

- excluding coverage for abortion services under health insurance, or failing to eliminate or reduce service fees for poor women and adolescents (see Chapter 3);

- failing to guarantee confidentiality and privacy, including for treatment of abortion complications (see Chapter 3);

- requiring women to provide the names of practitioners before providing them with treatment for complications from illegal abortion;

- restrictive interpretation of legal grounds.

These barriers contribute to unsafe abortion because they:

- deter women from seeking care and providers from delivering services within the formal health system;

- cause delay in access to services, which may result in denial of services due to gestational limits on the legal grounds;

- create complex and burdensome administrative procedures;

- increase the costs of accessing abortion services;

- limit the availability of services and their equitable geographic distribution.

Details of selected policy barriers follow.

4.2.2.1 Access to information

Access to information is a key determinant of safe abortion. Criminal laws, including on the provision of abortion-related information, and the stigmatization of abortion deter many women from requesting information from their regular health-care providers about legal services. Women may prefer not to consult their regular health-care providers, or to seek care outside their communities.

Many women and health-care providers (as well as police and court officers) do not know what the law allows with regard to abortion (*50, 51*). For instance, in a country where abortion is permitted up to 20 weeks of pregnancy to protect a woman's heath and for contraceptive failure, a survey revealed that more than 75% of married women and men were not aware that abortion was legal in these circumstances (*52*). Public health policies or regulations may contain special provisions that clarify how to interpret an abortion law. In many countries, however, no formal interpretation or enabling regulation exists (*53*). The fear of violating a law produces a chilling effect. Women are deterred from seeking services within the formal health sector. Health-care professionals tend to be overly cautious when deciding whether the legal grounds for abortion are met, thereby denying women services to which they are lawfully entitled. In other cases, there is inadequate or conflicting information, for instance, about appropriate dosages of drugs for medical abortion.

- The provision of information about safe, legal abortion is crucial to protect women's health and their human rights. States should decriminalize the provision of information related to legal abortion and should provide clear guidance on how legal grounds for abortion are to be interpreted and applied, as well as information on how and where to access lawful services. Legislators,

judges, prosecutors and policy-makers also need to understand the human rights and health dimensions of legal access to safe abortion services, made available through training or other appropriately targeted information.

4.2.2.2 Third-party authorization

The requirement for partner or parental authorization may deter women from seeking safe, legal services (*54*). Access to care may also be unduly delayed by burdensome procedures of medical authorization, especially where required specialists or hospital committees are inaccessible. The requirement for authorization by spouse, parent or hospital authorities may violate the right to privacy and women's access to health care on the basis of equality of men and women (*8,16*). Negotiating authorization procedures disproportionately burdens poor women, adolescents, those with little education, and those subjected to, or at risk of, domestic conflict and violence, creating inequality in access. Parental authorization – often based on an arbitrary age limit – denies the recognition of evolving capacities of young women (*55*).

- Third-party authorization should not be required for women to obtain abortion services. To protect the best interests and welfare of minors, and taking into consideration their evolving capacities, policies and practices should encourage, but not require, parents' engagement through support, information and education (see also Chapter 3).

4.2.2.3 Provision of essential medicines

Medical methods of abortion may be unavailable due to the lack of regulatory approval or registration for essential medicines. Both mifepristone and misoprostol have been included on the *WHO model list of essential medicines* since 2005 (*56, 57*), yet many countries have not yet registered the drugs or placed them on their national list of essential drugs. Sometimes legal restrictions may also be placed on the distribution of medicines after their approval.

- Registration and distribution of adequate supplies of drugs for medical abortion (see Chapter 3) are essential for improving the quality of abortion services, for any legal indication. Access to essential medicines is also necessary to avoid injury to women's health caused by use of unregistered drugs purchased through channels that are uncontrolled for quality.

4.2.2.4 Regulation of facilities and providers

Restrictions on the range of providers (e.g. gynaecologists only) or facilities (e.g. tertiary level only) that are legally authorized to provide abortion reduce the availability of services and their equitable geographic distribution, requiring women to travel greater distances for care, thereby raising costs and delaying access (58).

- The regulation of facilities and providers should be evidence-based to protect against over-medicalized, arbitrary or otherwise unreasonable requirements. Facility and provider regulation should be based on criteria currently required for provision of safe abortion care (see Chapter 3). Vacuum aspiration and the medical methods recommended in Chapter 2 can be safely provided at primary health-care level by midlevel providers (59, 60). The regulation of providers and facilities should be directed to ensuring that WHO-recommended methods can be provided both safely and efficiently.

4.2.2.5 Conscientious objection

Health-care professionals sometimes exempt themselves from abortion care on the basis of conscientious objection to the procedure, while not referring the woman to an abortion provider. In the absence of a readily available abortion-care provider, this practice can delay care for women in need of safe abortion, which increases risks to their health and life. While the right to freedom of thought, conscience, and religion is protected by international human rights law, international human rights law also stipulates that freedom to manifest one's religion or beliefs might be subject to limitations necessary to protect the fundamental human rights of others (61). Therefore laws and regulations should not entitle providers and institutions to impede women's access to lawful health services (62).

- Health-care professionals who claim conscientious objection must refer the woman to another willing and trained provider in the same, or another easily accessible health-care facility, in accordance with national law. Where referral is not possible, the health-care professional who objects must provide abortion to save the woman's life or to prevent damage to her health. Health services should be organized in such a way as to ensure that an effective exercise of the freedom of conscience of health professionals in the professional context does not prevent patients from obtaining access to services to which they are entitled under the applicable legislation.

4.2.2.6 Waiting periods

Mandatory waiting periods are often required by laws or regulations and/or administrative procedures imposed by facilities or individual providers. Mandatory waiting periods can have the effect of delaying care, which can jeopardize women's ability to access safe, legal abortion services and demeans women as competent decision-makers (24, 43).

- States and other providers of health services should ensure that abortion care is delivered in a manner that respects women as decision-makers. Waiting periods should not jeopardize women's access to safe, legal abortion services. States should consider eliminating waiting periods that are not medically required, and expanding services to serve all eligible women promptly.

4.2.2.7 Censoring, withholding or intentionally misrepresenting health-related information

Women have a right to be fully informed of their options for health care by properly trained personnel, including information about the likely benefits and potential adverse effects of proposed procedures and available alternatives (8). Censoring, withholding or intentionally misrepresenting information about abortion services can result in a lack of access to services or delays, which increase health risks for women. Provision of information is an essential part of good-quality abortion services (see Box 4.2 and also see Chapter 2 "Information and couselling").

Information must be complete, accurate and easy to understand, and be given in a way that facilitates

a woman being able to freely give her fully informed consent, respects her dignity, guarantees her privacy and confidentiality and is sensitive to her needs and perspectives (8).

- States should refrain from limiting access to means of maintaining sexual and reproductive health, including censoring, withholding or intentionally misrepresenting health-related information (63).

4.2.2.8 Access to treatment for abortion complications

Health-care providers are obligated to provide life-saving medical care to any woman who suffers abortion-related complications, including treatment of complications from unsafe abortion, regardless of the legal grounds for abortion (19). However, in some cases, treatment of abortion complications is administered only on condition that the woman provides information about the person(s) who performed the illegal abortion. This has been considered torture and inhuman and degrading treatment (20).

BOX 4.2

Essential information for women

- Women have the right to decide freely and responsibly whether and when to have children without coercion, discrimination or violence.
- How pregnancy occurs, its signs and symptoms, and where to obtain a pregnancy test.
- How to prevent unintended pregnancy, including where and how to obtain contraceptive methods, including condoms.
- Where and how to obtain safe, legal abortion services and their cost.
- The details of legal limitations on the maximum gestational age when abortion can be obtained.
- That abortion is a very safe procedure but the risk of complications increases with increasing gestational age.
- How to recognize complications of miscarriage and unsafe abortion, the life-saving importance of seeking treatment immediately, and when and where to obtain services.

- The practice of extracting confessions from women seeking emergency medical care as a result of illegal abortion, and the legal requirement for doctors and other health-care personnel to report cases of women who have undergone abortion, must be eliminated. States have an obligation to provide immediate and unconditional treatment to anyone seeking emergency medical care (*19, 20, 41*).

4.2.2.9 Restrictive interpretation of laws on abortion

The respect, protection and fulfilment of human rights require that governments ensure abortion services that are allowable by law are accessible in practice (*10, 64*). Institutional and administrative mechanisms should be in place and should protect against unduly restrictive interpretations of legal grounds. These mechanisms should allow service provider and facility administrator decisions to be reviewed by an independent body, should take into consideration the views of the pregnant woman, and should provide timely resolution of review processes (*64*).

4.3. Creating an enabling environment

An enabling environment is needed to ensure that every woman who is legally eligible has ready access to safe abortion care. Policies should be geared to respecting, protecting and fulfilling the human rights of women, to achieving positive health outcomes for women, to providing good-quality contraceptive information and services, and to meeting the particular needs of groups such as poor women, adolescents, rape survivors and women living with HIV. The respect, protection, and fulfilment of human rights require that comprehensive regulations and policies be in place and they address all elements listed in Section 4.2.2, to ensure that abortion is safe and accessible. Existing policies should be examined to ascertain where there are gaps and where improvements are needed (see also Chapter 3).

Policies should aim to:

- respect, protect and fulfil the human rights of women, including women's dignity, autonomy and equality;

- promote and protect the health of women, as a state of complete physical, mental and social well-being;

- minimize the rate of unintended pregnancy by providing good-quality contraceptive information and services, including a broad range of contraceptive methods, emergency contraception and comprehensive sexuality education;

- prevent and address stigma and discrimination against women who seek abortion services or treatment for abortion complications;

- reduce maternal mortality and morbidity due to unsafe abortion, by ensuring that every woman entitled to legal abortion care can access safe and timely services including post-abortion contraception;

- meet the particular needs of women belonging to vulnerable and disadvantaged groups, such as poor women, adolescents, single women, refugees and displaced women, women living with HIV, and survivors of rape.

While countries differ in prevailing national health system conditions and constraints on available resources, all countries can take immediate and targeted steps to elaborate comprehensive polices that expand access to sexual and reproductive health services, including safe abortion care.

References

1. Ahman E, Shah IH. New estimates and trends regarding unsafe abortion mortality. *International Journal of Gynecology and Obstetrics,* 2011, 115:121–126.

2. *Global burden of disease 2004 update.* Geneva: World Health Organization, 2008.

3. *Unsafe abortion: global and regional estimates of the incidence of unsafe abortion and associated mortality in 2008*, 6th ed. Geneva, World Health Organization, 2011.

4. Singh S. Hospital admissions resulting from unsafe abortion: estimates from 13 developing countries. *Lancet*, 2006, 368:1887–1892.

5. Shah I, Ahman E. Unsafe abortion: global and regional incidence, trends, consequences and challenges. *Journal of Obstetrics and Gynaecology Canada*, 2009, 31:1149–1158.

6. *Key actions for the further implementation of the Programme of Action of the International Conference on Population and Development, adopted by the twenty-first special session of the General Assembly, New York, 30 June–2 July 1999.* New York, United Nations, 1999.

7. *Safe abortion: technical and policy guidance for health systems*. Geneva, World Health Organization, 2003.

8. Committee on the Elimination of Discrimination against Women. *General recommendation no. 24: Women and health (article 12).* United Nations, 1999.

9. Human Rights Committee. *General comment no. 28: equality of rights between men and women (article 3)*, 20 March 2000. United Nations; Human Rights Committee. *Concluding observations: Ecuador,* 18 August 1998. United Nations; Human Rights Committee. *Concluding observations: Guatemala,* 27 August 2001. United Nations; Human Rights Committee. *Concluding observations: Poland,* 2 December 2004. United Nations. Human Rights Committee. *Concluding observations: Madagascar,* 11 May 2007. United Nations, Human Rights Committee. *Concluding observations: Chile,* 18 May 2007. United Nations; Human Rights Committee. *Concluding observations: Colombia*, 26 May 2004. United Nations; Human Rights Committee. *Karen Noella Llantoy Huaman v. Peru,* Communication no. 1153/2003, UN Doc. CCPR/C/85/D/1153/2003, 2005; Committee on the Elimination of Discrimination against Women, *Concluding observations: Colombia,* 5 February 1999. United Nations; Committee on the Elimination of Discrimination against Women, *Concluding comments: Nicaragua,* 2 February 2007. United Nations; Committee on the Elimination of Discrimination against Women. *Concluding comments: Brazil,* 10 August 2007. United Nations; Committee on Economic Social and Cultural Rights. *Concluding observations: Nepal,* 24 September 2001. United Nations; Committee on Economic, Social and Cultural Rights. *Concluding observations: Costa Rica,* 22 April 2008. United Nations; Committee on the Rights of the Child. *Concluding observations: Chile,* 23 April 2007. United Nations; *Protocol to the African Charter on Human and Peoples' Rights on the Rights of Women in Africa,* adopted 11 July 2003, Article 14.2. Maputo, African Commission on Human and People's Rights.

10. Committee on Economic Social and Cultural Rights. *Concluding observations: Malta,* 4 December 2004. United Nations; Committee on Economic Social and Cultural Rights. *Concluding observations: Monaco,* 13 June 2006. United Nations; Committee on the Elimination of Discrimination against Women. *General recommendation no. 24: Women and health* (article 12). United Nations; Committee on the Elimination of Discrimination against Women. *Concluding observations: Colombia,* 5 February 1999. United Nations; Committee on the Elimination of Discrimination against Women. *Concluding comments: Dominican Republic,* 18 August 2004. United Nations; *Protocol to the African Charter on Human and Peoples' Rights on the Rights of Women in Africa,* adopted 11 July 2003, Article 14.2. Maputo, African Commission on Human and People's Rights.

11. Committee on Economic, Social and Cultural Rights. *Concluding observations; Nepal,* 29 August 2001. United Nations; Committee on Economic Social and Cultural Rights. *Concluding observations: Malta,* 4 December 2004. United Nations; Committee on Economic, Social and Cultural Rights, *Concluding observations: Chile,* 1 December 2004. United Nations; Committee on Economic Social and Cultural Rights. *Concluding observations: Monaco,* 13 June 2006. United Nations; Committee on Economic, Social and Cultural Rights. *Concluding observations: Costa Rica,* 22 April 2008; United Nations; Committee on the Elimination of Discrimination against Women. *Concluding comments: Colombia,* 5 February 1999. United Nations; Committee on the Elimination of Discrimination against Women. *Concluding comments: Sri Lanka,* 1 February 2002. United Nations; Committee on the Elimination of Discrimination against Women. *Concluding comments: Honduras,* 10 August 2007. United Nations; Committee on the Elimination of Discrimination against Women. *L.C. v. Peru,* CEDAW/C/50/D/22/2009, 4 November 2011. United Nations; Committee on the Rights of the Child. *Concluding observations: Chile,* 23 April 2007; *Protocol to the African Charter on Human and Peoples' Rights on the Rights of Women in Africa,* adopted 11 July 2003, Article 14.2. Maputo, African Commission on Human and People's Rights.

12. Committee on the Elimination of Discrimination against Women. *Concluding comments: Colombia,* 5 February 1999, United Nations; Committee on the Elimination of Discrimination against Women. *Concluding comments: Mauritius,* 17 March 2006. United Nations; Committee on the Elimination of Discrimination against Women. *Concluding comments: Chile.* 25 August 2006. United Nations; Committee on the Elimination of Discrimination against Women, *Concluding comments: Nicaragua,* 2 February 2007. United Nations; Committee on the Elimination of Discrimination against Women. *Concluding comments: Brazil,* 10 August 2007; United Nations; Committee on the Elimination of Discrimination against Women. *Concluding comments: Liechtenstein,* 10 August 2007. United Nations. Committee on the Elimination of Discrimination against Women, *Concluding comments: Honduras,* 10 August 2007. United Nations; Human Rights Committee. *Concluding observations: El Salvador,* 18 November 2010. United Nations; Human Rights Committee. *Concluding observations: Guatemala,* 27 August 2001. United Nations.

13. Committee on the Elimination of Discrimination against Women. *General recommendation no. 24: Women and health* (article 12). United Nations, 1999; Committee on the Elimination of Discrimination against Women, *Concluding comments: Honduras,* 10 August 2007. United Nations; Committee on the Elimination of Discrimination against Women, *Concluding observations: Nicaragua,* 2 February 2007. United Nations; Committee on the Rights of the Child, *General comment no. 4 Adolescent health and development in the context of the Convention on the Rights of the Child.* United Nations, 2003; Committee on the Rights of the Child, *Concluding observations: Chile,* 23 April 2007. United Nations. *Protocol to the African Charter on Human and Peoples' Rights on the Rights of Women in Africa,,* adopted 11 July 2003, Article 14.2. Maputo, African Commission on Human and People's Rights.

14. Committee on the Elimination of Discrimination against Women. *General recommendation no. 24: Women and health* (article 12). United Nations, 1999.

15. Committee on Economic Social and Cultural Rights. *General comment no. 14: The right to the highest attainable standard of health* (article 12) United Nations, 2000; Committee on the Rights of the Child. *General comment no. 4 Adolescent health and development in the context of the Convention on the Rights of the Child.* 01 July 2003. United Nations; European Court of Human Rights. *Case of Tysiac v. Poland.* Council of Europe, 2007 (Application no. 5410/03); European Court of Human Rights. *Case of Open Door Counselling and Dublin Well Woman v. Ireland*, 1992, Series A, no. 246. Council of Europe.

16. Human Rights Committee. *General comment no. 28: equality of rights between men and women* (article 3). United Nations 2000; Committee on the Elimination of Discrimination against Women. *General recommendation no. 24: Women and health* (article 12). United Nations, 1999.

17. Committee on the Elimination of Discrimination against Women. *General recommendation no. 24: Women and health* (article 12). United Nations, 1999; Committee on the Elimination of Discrimination against Women. *Concluding comments: Colombia.* United Nations, 1999; Committee on the Elimination of Discrimination against Women, *Concluding comments: Nicaragua,* 2 February 2007. United Nations; Human Rights Committee *Concluding observations: Zambia,* 9 August 2007. United Nations; European Court of Human Rights, *R.R. v. Poland*, App. No. 27617/04, Eur. Ct. H.R, Council of Europe, 2011.

18. Committee on the Elimination of Discrimination against Women. *L.C. v. Peru,* CEDAW/C/50/D/22/2009, 4 November 2011. United Nations; European Court of Human Rights. *Tysiąc v. Poland*, App. no. 5410/03. Council of Europe, 2007; European Court of Human Rights. *A.B.C. v. Ireland*, App. no. 25579/05. Council of Europe, 2004.

19. Committee against Torture. *Concluding observations on Chile,* 14 June 2004. United Nations; Committee on the Elimination of Discrimination against Women, *Concluding comments: Sri Lanka,* 1 February 2002. United Nations; Committee on the Elimination of Discrimination against Women, *Concluding comments: Mauritius,* 17 March 2006. United Nations; Committee on the Elimination of Discrimination against Women. *Concluding comments: Chile,* 25 August 2006. United Nations; Committee on the Elimination of Discrimination against Women. *Concluding comments: Brazil,* 10 August 2007. United Nations; Committee on the Elimination of Discrimination against Women, *Concluding observations: Honduras,* 10 August 2007. United Nations.

20. Committee against Torture *Concluding observations on Chile,* 14 June 2004. United Nations.

21. Sedgh G, et al. Induced abortion: incidence and trends worldwide from 1995 to 2008. *Lancet,* 2012, 379:625–632.

22. Levine PB, Staiger D. Abortion policy and fertility outcomes: the Eastern European experience. *Journal of Law and Economics,* 2004, XLVII:223–243.

23. Grimes D et al. Unsafe abortion: the preventable pandemic. *Lancet*, 2006, 368:1908–1919.

24. Joyce et al. *The impact of state mandatory counselling and waiting period laws on abortion: a literature review.* New York, Guttmacher Institute, 2009.

25. Payne D. More British abortions for Irish women. *British Medical Journal*, 1999, 318(7176):77.

26. David HP. Soviet Union. In: *Abortion research: international experience.* HP David, ed. Lexington, MA, Lexington Books, 1974.

27. Serbanescu et al. The impact of recent policy changes on fertility, abortion, and contraceptive use in Romania. *Studies in Family Planning,* 1995, 26(2):76–87.

28. Zhirova IA et al. Abortion-related maternal mortality in the Russian Federation. *Studies in Family Planning,* 2004, 35(3):178–188.

29. *Millennium development goals in Russia: looking into the future*. Moscow, United Nations Development Programme, 2010.

30. Cook RJ, Dickens BM. Human rights dynamics of abortion law reform. *Human Rights Quarterly*, 2003, 25:1–59.

31. Boland R, Katzive L. Developments in laws on induced abortion: 1998–2007. *International Family Planning Perspectives*, 2008, 34:110–120.

32. Berer M. National laws and unsafe abortion: the parameters of change. *Reproductive Health Matters*, 2004, 12:1–8.

33. Bartlett LA et al. Risk factors for legal induced abortion-related mortality in the United States. *Obstetrics and Gynecology*, 2004, 103:729–737.

34. Jewkes R et al. The impact of age on the epidemiology of incomplete abortions in South Africa after legislative change. *British Journal of Obstetrics and Gynaecology*, 2004, 112:355–359.

35. *World Health Report 2008 – Primary health care: now more than ever*. Geneva, World Health Organization, 2008.

36. UN Department for Economic and Social Affairs. *World abortion policies 2011*. New York, Population Division, United Nations, 2011.

37. Singh S et al. *Abortion worldwide: a decade of uneven progress*. New York, Guttmacher Institute, 2009.

38. Oye-Adeniran BA, Umoh AV, Nnatu SNN. Complications of unsafe abortion: a case study and the need for abortion law reform in Nigeria. *Reproductive Health Matters*, 2002, 10:19–22.

39. Human Rights Committee. *Karen Noella Llantoy Huaman v. Peru*. Communication no. 1153/2003, UN Doc. CCPR/C/85/D/1153/2003, 2005. Committee on the Elimination of Discrimination against Women. *L.C. v. Peru*, CEDAW/C/50/D/22/2009, 4 November 2011. United Nations; Committee against Torture. *Concluding observations: Peru*, 16 May 2006. United Nations.

40. Constitution of the World Health Organization, 47th ed. Geneva, World Health Organization, 2009.

41. Human Rights Committee. *General comment no. 28: equality of rights between men and women (article 3)*. 20 March 2000. United Nations.

42. *Clinical management of rape survivors: developing protocols for use with refugees and internally displaced persons*. Geneva, World Health Organization, 2004.

43. Cook RJ, Dickens BM, Fathalla MF. *Reproductive health and human rights: integrating medicine, ethics and law*. Oxford, Oxford University Press, 2003.

44. Billings D et al. Constructing access to legal abortion services in Mexico City. *Reproductive Health Matters*, 2002, 10:87–95.

45. Villela WV, Oliveira Araujo M. Making legal abortion available in Brazil: partnership in practice. *Reproductive Health Matters*, 2000, 8:77–82.

46. Cook RJ, Ngwena CG. Women's access to health care: the legal framework. *International Journal of Gynecology and Obstetrics*, 2006, 94:216–225.

47. Cook RJ et al. Prenatal management of anencephaly. *International Journal of Gynecology and Obstetrics*, 2008, 102:304–308.

48. Becker D, Garcia SG, Larsen U. Knowledge and opinions about abortion law among Mexican youth. *International Family Planning Perspectives*, 2002, 28:205–213.

49. Goldman LA et al. Brazilian obstetrician-gynecologists and abortion: a survey of knowledge, opinions and practices. Reproductive Health, 2005, 2:10.

50. Jewkes R et al. Why are women still aborting outside designated facilities in metropolitan South Africa? *British Journal of Obstetrics and Gynaecology*, 2005, 112:1236–1242.

51. Morroni C, Myer L, Tibazarwa K. Knowledge of the abortion legislation among South African women: a cross-sectional study. *Reproductive Health*, 2006, 3:7.

52. Iyengar K, Iyengar SD. Elective abortion as a primary health service in rural India: experience with manual vacuum aspiration. *Reproductive Health Matters*, 2002, 10:54–63.

53. Cook RJ, Erdman JN, Dickens BM. Achieving transparency in implementing abortion laws. *International Journal of Gynecology and Obstetrics*, 2007, 99:157–161.

54. Mundigo A, Indriso C. *Abortion in the developing world*. London and New York, Zed Books, 1999.

55. Cook RJ, Erdman JN, Dickens BM. Respecting adolescents' confidentiality and reproductive and sexual choices. *International Journal of Gynecology and Obstetrics*, 2007, 92:182–187.

56. *WHO model list of essential medicines*, 16th ed. Geneva, World Health Organization, 2010.

57. PATH, World Health Organization, United Nations Population Fund. *Essential medicines for reproductive health: guiding principles for their inclusion on national medicines lists*. Seattle, WA, PATH, 2006.

58. Scott Jones B, Weitz TA. Legal barriers to second-trimester abortion provision and public health consequences. *American Journal of Public Health,* 2009, 99(4):623–630.

59. Warriner IK et al. Rates of complication in first-trimester manual vacuum abortion done by doctors and mid-level providers in South Africa and Vietnam: a randomised controlled equivalence trial. *Lancet*, 2006, 368:1965–1972

60. Warriner IK et al. Can midlevel health-care providers administer early medical abortion as safely and effectively as doctors? A randomised controlled equivalence trial in Nepal. *Lancet*, 2011, 377:1155–1161.

61. International Covenant on Civil and Political Rights, entry into force 23 March 1976, Article 18. United Nations.

62. European Court of Human Rights, *Kontakt-information-Therapie and Hagen v. Austria*, 57 Eur. Ct. H.R. 81. Council of Europe, 1988.

63. Committee on Economic Social and Cultural Rights. *General comment no. 14: The right to the highest attainable standard of health* (article 12), 2000. United Nations.

64. Committee on the Elimination of Discrimination against Women, *L.C. v. Peru,* CEDAW/C/50/D/22/2009, 4 November 2011. United Nations; European Court of Human Rights. *Case of Tysiac v. Poland*. Application no. 5410/03. Council of Europe, 2007; *Paulina del Carmen Ramirez Jacinto, Mexico, Friendly Settlement, Report No. 21/07, Petition 161–01, 9 March 2007*. Inter-American Commission on Human Rights, 2007.

ANNEXES

ANNEX 1
Research gaps identified at the technical consultation

- The efficacy of lower doses (such as 600 µg) of misoprostol when used following mifepristone (200 mg) at earlier gestational ages or for certain routes of administration.

- Whether a benefit exists when a starting dose, higher than the repeat dose of misoprostol, is used during second-trimester medical abortion.

- Identification of the most effective combined regimen of medical abortion between 9 and 12 weeks of gestation.

- Identification of the interval between mifepristone and misoprostol that women prefer, given that the timing that achieves the highest efficacy for abortion is between 24 and 48 hours.

- Evaluation of whether cervical preparation has an effect on the pain experienced by women during surgical abortion.

- Evaluation of whether cervical preparation has an effect on surgical abortion complications in the late first trimester (9–12 weeks of gestation).

- The risks and benefits of cervical preparation, and whether they vary by provider experience level.

- Identification of whether the pharmacokinetics of carboprost are similar to those of gemeprost.

- Evaluation of algorithms for follow-up after medical and surgical abortion.

- Evaluation of the safety of contraceptive use (particularly IUDs, implants and injectables) following medical abortion.

- Evaluation of the safe period of delay after a septic abortion when an IUD may be inserted.

- Evaluation of the best pain-management options for both first- and second-trimester abortions, including the timing of their administration.

- Evaluation of the role of incentives to providers for provision of abortion, and whether it differentially affects access to abortion services.

- Identification of how women pay for abortions and whether this information can be used to provide more equitable services.

- Evaluation of the effect of Internet provision, telemedicine, social marketing and other similar services on the safe provision of, and access to abortion services.

ANNEX 2
Final GRADE questions and outcomes

1. When mifepristone is not available, what is the recommended method of medical abortion up to 12 weeks of gestation?

   a. Outcome 1: failure to complete abortion

   b. Outcome 2: ongoing pregnancy

   c. Outcome 3: side-effects (overall, individual)

   d. Outcome 4: abortion interval from initiation of treatment

   e. Outcome 5: other procedure-related complications

2. What method of pain control should be used for surgical abortion up to 12–14 weeks of gestation?

   a. Outcome 1: effectiveness in decreasing procedural pain

   b. Outcome 2: side-effects (overall, individual)

   c. Outcome 3: complications related to pain-control methods

3. Should antibiotics be used to prevent post-abortion infection?

   a. Outcome 1: infection

   b. Outcome 2: side-effects (overall, individual)

   c. Outcome 3: complications

   d. Outcome 4: cost

4. What is the recommended medical regimen for abortion up to 12 weeks of gestation?[1]

   a. Outcome 1: failure to complete abortion

   b. Outcome 2: ongoing pregnancy

   c. Outcome 3: side-effects (overall, individual)

   d. Outcome 4: abortion interval from initiation of treatment

   e. Outcome 5: other procedure-related complications

5. What is the recommended method of abortion after 12 weeks of gestation?

   a. Outcome 1: failure to complete abortion

   b. Outcome 2: ongoing pregnancy

   c. Outcome 3: side-effects (overall, individual)

   d. Outcome 4: abortion interval from initiation of treatment

   e. Outcome 5: other procedure-related complications

6. How should incomplete abortion be treated?

   a. Outcome 1: failure to complete abortion

   b. Outcome 2: side-effects (overall, individual)

   c. Outcome 3: abortion interval from initiation of treatment

   d. Outcome 4: other procedure-related complications

7. What method of medical abortion should be used beyond 12 weeks of gestation?

   a. Outcome 1: complete abortion

   b. Outcome 2: side-effects (overall, individual)

   c. Outcome 3: procedure-related complications

   d. Outcome 4: abortion interval from initiation of treatment

8. How should cervical preparation prior to surgical abortion be accomplished?

   a. Outcome 1: successful cervical dilatation

   b. Outcome 2: degree (in mm) of cervical dilatation

   c. Outcome 3: patient acceptability

   d. Outcome 4: procedure duration

   e. Outcome 5: interval from treatment to completed abortion

   f. Outcome 6: side-effects (overall, individual)

   g. Outcome 7: complications

9. Who should receive cervical preparation prior to surgical abortion?

   a. Outcome 1: no need for further dilatation

   b. Outcome 2: degree (in mm) of cervical dilatation

   c. Outcome 3: patient preference

   d. Outcome 4: complications

10. What methods of pain control should be used for medical abortion?

   a. Outcome 1: side-effects (overall, individual)

   b. Outcome 2: complications

   c. Outcome 3: abortion interval from initiation of treatment

   d. Outcome 4: effectiveness in relieving procedural pain

11. Should pre-abortion ultrasound be recommended?

   a. Outcome 1: complications

   b. Outcome 2: failure to complete abortion

12. What method of surgical abortion should be used prior to 12 weeks of gestation?

   a. Outcome 1: failure to complete abortion

   b. Outcome 2: side-effects (overall, individual)

   c. Outcome 3: other procedure-related complications

13. Should women have routine follow-up following induced abortion?

   a. Outcome 1: complications

   b. Outcome 2: cost

   c. Outcome 3: patient acceptability

[1] Note that in the recommendations (Annex 5), this question was separated into two recommendations, based on gestational age <9 weeks and gestational age 9–12 weeks

ANNEX 3
Standard GRADE criteria for grading of evidence
See references *19–23*.

Domain	Grade	Characteristic
Study design	0	All randomized controlled trials
	−1	All observational studies
Study design limitations	0	Most of the pooled effect provided by studies, with low risk of bias
	−1	Most of the pooled effect provided by studies with moderate or high risk of bias
	−2	Most of the pooled effect provided by studies with moderate or high risk of bias
	Note:	*Low risk of bias*: no limitations or minor limitations
		Moderate risk of bias: serious limitations or potentially very serious limitations including unclear concealment of allocation or serious limitations, excluding limitations on randomization or concealment of allocation
		High risk of bias: limitations for randomization, concealment of allocation, including small blocked randomization (<10) or other very serious, crucial methodological limitations
Inconsistency	0	No severe heterogeneity ($I^2 < 60\%$ or $\chi^2 \geq 0.05$)
	−1	Severe, non-explained, heterogeneity ($I^2 \geq 60\%$ or $\chi^2 < 0.05$)
		If heterogeneity could be caused by publication bias or imprecision due to small studies, downgrade only for publication bias or imprecision (i.e. the same weakness should not be downgraded twice)
Indirectness	0	No indirectness
	−1	Presence of indirect comparison, population, intervention, comparator, or outcome
Imprecision	0	The confidence interval is precise according to the figure below suggested appreciable benefit — risk ratio — suggested appreciable harm precise imprecise 0.75 1.0 1.25 The total cumulative study population is not very small (i.e. sample size is more than 300 participants) and the total number of events is more than 30
	−1	One of the above-mentioned conditions is not fulfilled
	−2	The two above-mentioned are not fulfilled
	Note:	If the total number of events is less than 30 and the total cumulative sample size is appropriately large (e.g. above 3000 patients), consider not downgrading the evidence. If there are no events in both intervention and control groups, the quality of evidence in the specific outcome should be regarded as very low.
Publication bias	0	No evident asymmetry in the funnel plot or fewer than five studies to be plotted
	−1	Evident asymmetry in the funnel plot with at least five studies

ANNEX 4
Participants in the technical consultation

Dr Marijke Alblas
Clinician, health advocate
Independent medical consultant
Cape Town
South Africa

Ms Marge Berer
Health advocate
Editor
Reproductive Health Matters
London
United Kingdom of Great Britain and Northern Ireland

Dr Mohsina Bilgrami
Programme manager, policy-maker, health advocate
Managing Director
Marie Stopes Society
Karachi
Pakistan

Dr Paul Blumenthal
Clinician, researcher
Professor of Obstetrics and Gynecology
Stanford University School of Medicine
Stanford, CA
United States of America

Dr Lidia Casas-Becerra
Lawyer, researcher, health advocate
Professor of Law
Diego Portales Law School
Universidad Diego Portales
Santiago
Chile

Dr Laura Castleman
Clinician, programme manager
Medical Director
Ipas
Birmingham, MI
USA

Ms Jane Cottingham
Researcher, health advocate
Independent consultant in sexual and reproductive
health and rights
Carouge, GE
Switzerland

Dr Kelly Culwell
Clinician, health advocate, programme manager
Senior adviser
International Planned Parenthood Federation
London
United Kingdom of Great Britain and Northern Ireland

Dr Teresa Depiñeres
Researcher, clinician, programme manager
Senior Technical Advisor
Fundacion Orientame
Bogota
Colombia

Dr Joanna Erdman
Lawyer, researcher, health advocate
Adjunct Professor, Faculty of Law
University of Toronto
Ontario
Canada

Dr Aníbal Faúndes
Clinician, health advocate
Professor of Obstetrics and Gynaecology
State University of Campinas
Campinas, São Paulo
Brazil

Professor Mahmoud Fathalla
Clinician, researcher, health advocate
Assiut University
Assiut
Egypt

Dr Kristina Gemzell-Danielsson
Researcher, clinician, policy-maker
Professor of Obstetrics and Gynaecology
Karolinska University Hospital
Stockholm
Sweden

Dr Anna Glasier
Clinician, researcher
Lead Clinician, Sexual Health
NHS Lothian and University of Edinburgh
Edinburgh
Scotland

Dr Türkiz Gökgöl
Researcher, policy-maker, programme manager
Director of International Programs
The Susan Thompson Buffett Foundation
Omaha, NE
United States of America

Dr David Grimes
Methodologist, epidemiologist, researcher
Distinguished scientist
Family Health International
Durham, NC
United States of America

Dr Selma Hajri
Clinician, researcher
Consultant in reproductive health
Coordinator
African Network for Medical Abortion (ANMA)
Tunis
Tunisia

Dr Pak Chung Ho
Clinician, researcher
Professor of Obstetrics and Gynaecology
Queen Mary Hospital
Hong Kong
People's Republic of China

Dr Sharad Iyengar
Clinician, policy-maker
Chief Executive
Action Research & Training for Health
Udaipur
India

Ms Heidi Bart Johnston
Temporary Adviser
Reproductive Health and Rights Consultant
Wetzikon
Switzerland

Ms Bonnie Scott Jones
Lawyer, health advocate
Deputy Director
Center for Reproductive Rights
New York, NY
United States of America

Dr Vasantha Kandiah
Researcher
Consultant
Population and Family Planning Development Board
Kuala Lumpur
Malaysia

Dr Nguyen Duy Khe
Programme manager
Head, Mother and Child Healthcare Department
Ministry of Health
Hanoi
Viet Nam

Dr Chisale Mhango
Programme manager
Director, Reproductive Health Unit
Ministry of Health
Lilongwe
Malawi

Dr Suneeta Mittal
Clinician, researcher, health advocate
Head, Department of Obstetrics and Gynecology
All India Institute of Medical Sciences
Ansari Nagar, New Delhi
India

Dr Nuriye Ortayli
Clinician, programme manager
Senior Adviser
UNFPA
New York, NY
United States of America

Dr Mariana Romero
Researcher, health advocate
Associate researcher
CEDES
Buenos Aires
Argentina

Dr Helena von Hertzen
Researcher
Consultant
Concept Foundation
Geneva
Switzerland

Dr Beverly Winikoff
Methodologist, epidemiologist, researcher
President
Gynuity Health Projects
New York, NY
United States of America

Ms Patricia Ann Whyte
Temporary Adviser
Senior research fellow
Deakin Strategic Centre in Population Health
Faculty of Health, Deakin University
Victoria
Australia

Additional peer reviewers
Ms Rebecca Cook
Chair in International Human Rights Law
Faculty of Law
University of Toronto
Toronto, Ontario
Canada

Ms Laura Katsive
Program Officer
Wellspring Advisors, LLC
New York
United States of America

Dr Paul FA Van Look
Consultant in Sexual and Reproductive Health
Val d'Illiez
Switzerland

WHO regional advisers
Dr Khadiddiatou Mbaye, Regional Office for Africa
Dr Gunta Lazdane, Regional Office for Europe

WHO Secretariat
Dr Katherine Ba-Thike
Dr Dalia Brahmi
Dr Peter Fajans
Dr Bela Ganatra
Dr Emily Jackson
Dr Ronald Johnson
Dr Nathalie Kapp
Ms Eszter Kismodi
Dr Regina Kulier
Dr Michael Mbizvo
Dr Lale Say
Dr Iqbal Shah
Dr João Paulo Dias de Souza

Observers
Dr Mari Mathiesen
Member of the Management Board
Estonian Health Insurance Fund
Lembitu
Estonia

Dr Helvi Tarien
Head of Health Services Department
Estonian Health Insurance Fund
Lembitu
Estonia

ANNEX 5

Recommendations from the technical consultation for the second edition of *Safe abortion: technical and policy guidance for health systems*

Recommendation 1: surgical abortion up to gestational age 12 to 14 weeks

Vacuum aspiration is the recommended technique of surgical abortion for pregnancies of up to 12 to 14 weeks of gestation. The procedure should not be routinely completed by sharp curettage. Dilatation and sharp curettage (D&C), if still practised, should be replaced by vacuum aspiration.

(Strength of recommendation: strong)

Remarks

- Observational studies indicate that vacuum aspiration is associated with fewer complications than D&C; however, randomized controlled trials were underpowered to detect a difference in complication rates.

- No evidence supports the use of sharp curette checks (i.e. the use of sharp curettage to "complete" the abortion) following vacuum aspiration.

- The quality of the evidence based on randomized controlled trials is low to moderate.

Recommendation 2: medical abortion up to gestational age 9 weeks (63 days)

Recommendation 2.1

The recommended method for medical abortion is mifepristone followed by misoprostol.

(Strength of recommendation: strong)

Remarks

- Randomized controlled trials demonstrate superior effectiveness of the combined regimen (mifepristone followed by misoprostol) when compared with misoprostol used alone.

- The quality of the evidence based on randomized controlled trials is moderate.

Recommendation 2.2

Mifepristone should always be administered orally. The recommended dose is 200 mg.

(Strength of recommendation: strong)

Remarks

- Randomized controlled trials indicate that 200 mg of mifepristone is as efficacious as 600 mg.

- The quality of the evidence based on randomized controlled trials is moderate.

Recommendation 2.3

For vaginal, buccal or sublingual routes, the recommended dose of misoprostol is 800 μg. For oral administration, the recommended dose of misoprostol is 400 μg.

(Strength of recommendation: strong)

Remarks

- The efficacy of misoprostol may vary depending upon gestational age, the route of administration, or the frequency of dosing. Research is currently ongoing to determine in what clinical situations, if any, a lower dose of misoprostol might be used with comparable efficacy.

- The quality of the evidence based on randomized controlled trials is moderate.

Recommendation 2.4

Recommended dosages and routes of administration for mifepristone followed by misoprostol:

Mifepristone should always be administered orally. The recommended dose is 200 mg.

Administration of misoprostol is recommended 1 to 2 days (24 to 48 hours) following ingestion of mifepristone.

- For vaginal, buccal or sublingual routes, the recommended dose of misoprostol is 800 μg.

- For oral administration, the recommended dose of misoprostol is 400 μg.

- With gestations up to 7 weeks (49 days) misoprostol may be administered by vaginal, buccal, sublingual or oral routes. After 7 weeks of gestation, oral administration of misoprostol should not be used.

- With gestations up to 9 weeks (63 days) misoprostol can be administered by vaginal, buccal or sublingual routes.

(Strength of recommendation: strong)

Remarks

- Vaginal administration of misoprostol is recommended based on its higher effectiveness and lower rates of side-effects than other routes of administration; however, some women may prefer a non-vaginal route.

- The quality of the evidence based on randomized controlled trials is moderate.

Recommendation 2.5

Administration of misoprostol is recommended 1 to 2 days (24 to 48 hours) following ingestion of mifepristone.

(Strength of recommendation: strong)

Remark

- The quality of the evidence based on randomized controlled trials is moderate.

Recommendation 3: medical abortion for gestational age between 9 and 12 weeks (63 and 84 days)

The recommended method for medical abortion is 200 mg mifepristone administered orally followed 36 to 48 hours later by 800 μg misoprostol administered vaginally. Subsequent misoprostol doses should be 400 μg, administered either vaginally or sublingually, every 3 hours up to four further doses, until expulsion of the products of conception.

(Strength of recommendation: weak)

Remarks

- The regimen for medical abortion between 9 and 12 weeks of gestation is an area of ongoing research; this recommendation is likely to be affected as studies are completed.

- The quality of evidence based on one randomized controlled trial and one observational study is low.

Recommendation 4: medical abortion up to gestational age 12 weeks (84 days) *where mifepristone is not available*

The recommended method of medical abortion where mifepristone is not available is 800 µg of misoprostol administered by vaginal or sublingual routes. Up to three repeat doses of 800 µg can be administered at intervals of at least 3 hours, but for no longer than 12 hours.

(Strength of recommendation: strong)

Remarks

- Sublingual misoprostol is associated with higher rates of side-effects than vaginal administration. In nulliparous women, the sublingual route is also less efficacious when intervals greater than 3 hours between repeat doses are used.

- The quality of the evidence based on one randomized controlled trial is high.

- Mifepristone with misoprostol is more effective than misoprostol used alone, and is associated with fewer side-effects. Methotrexate combined with misoprostol, a regimen used in some areas but not recommended by WHO, is less effective than mifepristone with misoprostol, but is more effective than misoprostol used alone.

Recommendation 5: methods of abortion after gestational age 12 to 14 weeks (84 to 98 days)

Dilatation and evacuation (D&E) and medical methods (mifepristone and misoprostol; misoprostol alone) are both recommended methods for abortion for gestations over 12 to 14 weeks. Facilities should offer at least one, and preferably both, methods if possible, depending on provider experience and the availability of training.

(Strength of recommendation: strong)

Remarks

- Evidence for this question is limited by women's willingness to be randomized in clinical trials between surgical and medical methods of abortion.

- The quality of the evidence based on randomized controlled trials is low.

- A woman's choice of abortion method may be limited or not applicable if she has medical contraindications to one of the methods.

Recommendation 6: medical abortion after gestational age 12 weeks (84 days)

The recommended method for medical abortion is 200 mg mifepristone administered orally followed 36 to 48 hours later by repeated doses of misoprostol.

(Strength of recommendation: strong)

- With gestations between 12 and 24 weeks, the initial misoprostol dose following oral mifepristone administration may be either 800 µg administered vaginally or 400 µg administered orally. Subsequent misoprostol doses should be 400 µg, administered either vaginally or sublingually, every 3 hours up to four further doses.

– For pregnancies beyond 24 weeks, the dose of misoprostol should be reduced, due to the greater sensitivity of the uterus to prostaglandins, but the lack of clinical studies precludes specific dosing recommendations.

(Strength of recommendation: strong)

The recommended method of medical abortion where mifepristone is not available is 400 µg of misoprostol administered vaginally or sublingually, repeated every 3 hours for up to five doses.

(Strength of recommendation: strong)

Remarks

• An interval of less than 36 hours between administration of mifepristone and misoprostol is associated with a longer interval to abortion and higher rates of incomplete abortion.

• Ethacridine lactate is associated with a similar interval to abortion as regimens using misoprostol alone; studies have not compared the safety or efficacy of its use to that of combined mifepristone and misoprostol.

• Women with a uterine scar have a very low (0.28%) risk of uterine rupture during medical abortion in the second trimester.

• When using misoprostol alone in nulliparous women, vaginal administration of misoprostol is more effective than sublingual administration.

• The quality of the evidence based on randomized controlled trials is low to moderate.

Recommendation 7: cervical preparation prior to surgical abortion up to gestational age 12 to 14 weeks (84 to 98 days)

Recommendation 7.1

Prior to surgical abortion, cervical preparation is recommended for all women with a pregnancy over 12 to 14 weeks of gestation. Its use may be considered for women with a pregnancy of any gestational age.

(Strength of recommendation: strong)

Remarks

• Consideration should be given to the increase in time and side-effects, including pain, vaginal bleeding and precipitous abortion, associated with cervical preparation if used at gestational ages <12 to 14 weeks.

• Lack of availability of cervical preparation should not limit access to abortion services.

• The quality of the evidence based on randomized controlled trials is low.

Recommendation 7.2

Any one of these methods of cervical preparation before surgical abortion in the first trimester is recommended:

– oral mifepristone 200 mg (24 to 48 hours in advance); or

– misoprostol 400 µg administered sublingually, 2 to 3 hours prior to the procedure; or

– misoprostol 400 µg administered vaginally 3 hours prior to the procedure; or

– laminaria placed intracervically 6 to 24 hours prior to the procedure.

(Strength of recommendation: strong)

Remarks

- Cost, local availability of and training in the use of cervical preparatory methods will affect the choice of method to use.

- The quality of the evidence based on randomized controlled trials is low to moderate.

Recommendation 8: cervical preparation prior to surgical abortion for gestational age ≥14 weeks (98 days)

Recommendation 8.1

All women undergoing dilatation and evacuation (D&E) with a pregnancy over 14 weeks of gestation should receive cervical preparation prior to the procedure.

(Strength of recommendation: strong)

Remark

- The quality of the evidence based on randomized controlled trials is low to moderate.

Recommendation 8.2

The recommended methods of cervical preparation prior to dilatation and evacuation (D&E) after 14 weeks of gestation are osmotic dilators or misoprostol.

(Strength of recommendation: strong)

Remarks

- Osmotic dilators reduce procedure time and the need for further dilatation when compared with use of misoprostol. The effect of misoprostol prior to D&E for pregnancies of gestational age over 20 weeks has not been the subject of clinical research.

- The quality of the evidence based on randomized controlled trials is moderate.

Recommendation 9: follow-up after induced abortion

There is no medical need for a routine follow-up visit following uncomplicated surgical abortion or medical abortion using mifepristone followed by misoprostol. However, women should be advised that additional services are available to them if needed or desired.

(Strength of recommendation: strong)

Remarks

- Women must be adequately informed regarding symptoms of ongoing pregnancy and other medical reasons, such as prolonged heavy bleeding or fever, to return for follow-up.

- Alternative follow-up strategies to in-clinic visits after first-trimester medical abortion are the subject of ongoing research.

- The quality of the evidence based on observational studies and indirect evidence is low.

Recommendation 10: treatment of incomplete abortion

If uterine size at the time of treatment is equivalent to a pregnancy of gestational age 13 weeks or less, either vacuum aspiration or treatment with misoprostol is recommended for women with incomplete abortion. The recommended regimen of misoprostol is a single dose given either sublingually (400 µg) or orally (600 µg).

(Strength of recommendation: strong)

Remarks

- Expectant management of incomplete abortion can be as effective as misoprostol, but the process takes more time. The decision for treatment or expectant management of incomplete abortion should be based on the clinical condition of the woman and her preferences for treatment.

- This recommendation is extrapolated from research conducted in women with reported spontaneous abortion. Missed abortion is a different condition from incomplete abortion following either spontaneous or induced abortion.

- Based on the recommendation for surgical abortion through the first trimester, vacuum aspiration may also be used in women with a uterine size of 14 weeks of gestation.

- Misoprostol may also be used vaginally. Studies of vaginal misoprostol have used doses ranging from 400 µg to 800 µg, and comparative dosing trials have not been reported.

- The quality of the evidence based on randomized controlled trials is low.

Recommendation 11: antibiotic prophylaxis for induced abortion

All women having surgical abortion, regardless of their risk of pelvic inflammatory infection, should receive appropriate prophylactic antibiotics pre- or peri-operatively.

(Strength of recommendation: strong)

For women having medical abortion, routine use of prophylactic antibiotics is not recommended.

(Strength of recommendation: strong)

Remarks

- Lack of antibiotics should not limit access to abortion services.

- Single-dose administration of nitroimidazoles, tetracyclines or penicillins has been shown to be effective.

- The quality of the evidence based on randomized controlled trials for surgical abortion is moderate. The quality of the evidence based on one observational trial for medical abortion is very low; for surgical abortion it is moderate.

Recommendation 12: ultrasound use prior to induced abortion

Use of routine pre-abortion ultrasound scanning is not necessary.

(Strength of recommendation: strong)

Remark

- The quality of the evidence based on a randomized controlled trial and observational studies is very low.

Recommendation 13: contraception following abortion

Women may start hormonal contraception at the time of surgical abortion, or as early as the time of administration of the first pill of a medical abortion regimen.

(Strength of recommendation: strong)

Following medical abortion, an IUD may be inserted when it is reasonably certain that the woman is no longer pregnant.

Remarks

- Initiation of hormonal contraception during medical abortion prior to expulsion of the pregnancy has not been the subject of clinical trials.

- The quality of evidence based on randomized controlled trials is very low.

Recommendation 14: pain management during abortion

All women should routinely be offered pain medication (e.g. non-steroidal anti-inflammatory drugs) during both medical and surgical abortions.

(Strength of recommendation: strong)

General anaesthesia is not routinely recommended for vacuum aspiration abortion or D&E.

(Strength of recommendation: strong)

Remarks

- Medication for pain management for both medical and surgical abortions should always be offered, and provided without delay to women who desire it. In most cases, analgesics, local anaesthesia and/or conscious sedation supplemented by verbal reassurance are sufficient, although the need for pain management increases with gestational age.

- The timing of pain medication administration has been inadequately and poorly studied, which precludes making recommendations about specific regimen(s); however, providing pain management is an important part of safe abortion care.

- Intravenous narcotics and/or tranquillizers and paracervical block are widely used, despite being inadequately studied.

- Non-steroidal anti-inflammatory drugs have demonstrated effectiveness in decreasing pain; in contrast, paracetamol has been shown to be ineffective at decreasing pain associated with surgical or medical abortion.

- Some women may require additional narcotic pain medication, especially during second-trimester abortion.

- The use of regional anaesthesia during medical abortion for pregnancies of gestational age over 12 weeks has not been the subject of clinical trials.

- General anaesthesia is associated with higher rates of side-effects and adverse events than other methods of pain management.

- The quality of the evidence based on randomized controlled trials is low.

ANNEX 6
Post-abortion medical eligibility for contraceptive use[1]

Table A1. Summary table of post-abortion medical eligibility recommendations for hormonal contraceptives, intrauterine devices and barrier contraceptive methods											
Post-abortion condition	COC	CIC	Patch & vaginal ring	POP	DMPA, NET-EN	LNG/ ETG implants	Copper-bearing IUD	LNG-releasing IUD	Condom	Spermicide	Diaphragm
First trimester	1	1	1	1	1	1	1	1	1	1	1
Second trimester	1	1	1	1	1	1	2	2	1	1	1
Immediate post-septic abortion	1	1	1	1	1	1	4	4	1	1	1

CIC, combined injectable contraceptive; COC, combined oral contraceptive; DMPA/NET-EN, progestogen-only injectables: depot medroxyprogesterone acetate/norethisterone enanthate; IUD, intrauterine device; LNG/ETG, progestogen-only implants: levenorgestrel/etonorgestrel; POP, progesterone-only pill.

Definition of categories

- *1*: a condition for which there is no restriction for the use of the contraceptive method.

- *2*: a condition where the advantages of using the method generally outweigh the theoretical or proven risks.

- *3*: a condition where the theoretical or proven risks usually outweigh the advantages of using the method.

- *4*: a condition which represents an unacceptable health risk if the contraceptive method is used.

---

[1] Based on *Medical eligibility criteria for contraceptive use*, 4th ed. Geneva, World Health Organization, 2009.

Table A2. Post-abortion medical eligibility recommendations for female surgical sterilization

Post-abortion condition	Female surgical sterilization
Uncomplicated	A
Post-abortal sepsis or fever	D
Severe post-abortal haemorrhage	D
Severe trauma to the genital tract; cervical or vaginal tear at the time of abortion	D
Uterine perforation	S
Acute haematometra	D

Definition of categories

- *A = (accept):* there is no reason to deny sterilization to a person with this condition.

- *C = (caution)*: the procedure is normally conducted in a routine setting, but with extra preparation and precautions.

- *D = (delay)*: the procedure is delayed until the condition is evaluated and/or corrected; alternative temporary methods of contraception should be provided.

- *S = (special)*: the procedure should be undertaken in a setting with an experienced surgeon and staff, and equipment is needed to provide general anaesthesia, and other back-up medical support. For these conditions, the capacity to decide on the most appropriate procedure and anaesthesia regimen is also needed. Alternative temporary methods of contraception should be provided, if referral is required or there is otherwise any delay.

ANNEX 7
Core international and regional human rights treaties

Table A3. Core international human rights treaties	
International human rights treaty (date of entry into force)	**Treaty monitoring body**
International Convention on the Elimination of All Forms of Racial Discrimination (ICERD) (1969)	Committee on the Elimination of Racial Discrimination
International Covenant on Economic, Social and Cultural Rights (ICESCR) (1976)	Committee on Economic, Social and Cultural Rights
International Covenant on Civil and Political Rights (ICCPR) (1976)	Human Rights Committee
Convention on the Elimination of Discrimination Against Women (CEDAW) (1981)	Committee on the Elimination of Discrimination Against Women
Convention against Torture and Other Cruel, Inhuman or Degrading Treatment or Punishment (CAT) (1987)	Committee Against Torture
Convention on the Rights of the Child (CRC) (1990)	Committee on the Rights of the Child
International Convention on the Protection of the Rights of all Migrant Workers and Members of their Families (2003)	Committee on Migrant Workers
Convention on the Rights of Persons with Disabilities (CRPD) (2008)	Committee on the Rights of Persons with Disabilities

Table A4. Regional human rights treaties

Regional human rights treaty (date of entry into force)	Treaty monitoring body
American Declaration on the Rights and Duties of Man (1948)	Inter-American Commission on Human Rights
Convention for the Protection of Human Rights and Fundamental Freedoms (as amended by Protocols 1, 4, 6, 7, 12 and 13) (1953)	European Court of Human Rights
American Convention on Human Rights (1978)	Inter-American Commission on Human Rights
African Charter on Human and Peoples' Rights (1986)	African Commission on Human and Peoples' Rights
Inter-American Convention on the Prevention, Punishment and Eradication of Violence Against Women ("Convention of Belem do Para") (1994)	Inter-American Commission on Human Rights
European Social Charter (1961)/Revised European Social Charter (1996)	European Committee on Social Rights
African Charter on the Rights and Welfare of the Child (1999)	African Committee of Experts on the Rights and Welfare of the Child
Additional Protocol to the American Convention on Human Rights in the Area of Economic, Social and Cultural Rights ("Protocol of San Salvador") (1999)	Inter-American Commission on Human Rights
Protocol to the African Charter on Human and Peoples' Rights on the Rights of Women in Africa (2005)	African Commission on Human and Peoples' Rights
Arab Charter on Human Rights (2008)	Arab Human Rights Committee
Charter of Fundamental Rights of the European Union (2009)	General Court/European Court of Justice